# Fibromyalgia
# and Muscle Pain
## Your Guide to Self-Treatment

# Fibromyalgia
# and
# Muscle Pain

## Your Guide to
## Self-Treatment

**Leon Chaitow, ND, DO**

Conari
Press

This edition first published in 2015 by Conari Press
an imprint of Red Wheel/Weiser, LLC
With offices at:
665 Third Street, Suite 400
San Francisco, CA 94107
www.redwheelweiser.com
Sign up for our newsletter and special offers by going to
www.redwheelweiser.com/newsletter.

ISBN: 978-1-57324-656-9
Library of Congress Cataloging-in-Publication Data available upon request

Cover design by Jim Warner
Text design by Valerie Cooper
Typeset in Chaparral Pro & Univers

Printed in the United States of America
MG
10 9 8 7 6 5 4 3 2 1

# Contents

# Questionnaire Index

# Foreword

It is difficult to approach a new book by Dr. Leon Chaitow without some measure of bias. The exceptional merit of his previous books leaves one expecting the same from each new one. This biased expectation is fully justified by this new edition of *Fibromyalgia and Muscle Pain*. With the clarity that is a hallmark of Chaitow's books, he makes these complex disorders easy to understand. At the same time, he provides the reader with an array of practical, self-help methods of treatment. Chaitow also leaves the reader with the invaluable awareness that any self-help method works best as part of an integrated approach to treatment. This integrated approach is vital to most patients' recovery from fibromyalgia and muscle pain, and having long championed the approach, Chaitow teaches it as few other writers can. This third edition of *Fibromyalgia and Muscle Pain* is essential not only for those who want to free themselves from these disorders, but also for loved ones and clinicians who want to help them do so.

Dr. John C. Lowe
Board Certified: American Academy of Pain Management
Director of Research: Fibromyalgia Research Foundation

# Introduction:
# The Big Picture

Fibromyalgia and other chronic muscle pain and fatigue syndromes are complex. Before investigating what is known about the causes and the possible solutions to these problems, an explanation is needed as to how the body becomes unwell, and how it can be helped to recover.

To do this, some simple examples will be used and the reader is asked to refer to the first few pages of Chapter 6, particularly to the diagram and notes associated with Figure 6.1 (page 123). This deals with the biochemical, biomechanical and psychological 'load' with which your body, and mind, are coping, and what happens when the load is too heavy, our adaptive processes fail and symptoms start.

Let's start with a few basic examples.

If you cut yourself, unless the wound is infected the cut will heal over a period of a few days. You know this, and you trust your body to do the repair work necessary. All you have to do is avoid getting the wound dirty and try not to aggravate it, as repair takes place – *automatically*.

More simplistically still, if you play a sport or dig the garden before you have acclimatized your muscles to the efforts involved, you will be stiff and will ache for a day or so afterwards. You *know* that this will pass as normal repair mechanisms sort out the overload and minor muscle damage.

If you catch a cold, and you are in reasonable health, you *know* that the cold will get better, in a week or two. There are many things you can do to make yourself more comfortable during the recovery phase, but not much you can do to speed up the process. But you do know that you will get better, and that the healing process is automatic.

In the same way, if you eat contaminated food, you may develop diarrhoea or vomit. Neither symptom is pleasant, but both are designed to get whatever is undesirable out of your system as fast as possible. Usually, with a little rest and a lot of liquid, recovery is rapid and complete. The body will heal itself.

In fact, most illnesses get better on their own (research suggests well over 90 per cent of infections get better without any treatment), but few of the symptoms associated with getting well are enjoyable (fever, diarrhoea, inflammation, etc.).

But headaches do go away, cuts do heal, bones do mend, and colds and most infections are taken care of by our amazing defence and repair systems. There is a constant tendency towards 'wellness', but the processes involved are not always comfortable.

Together, the self-repair, self-regulating and self-balancing systems of the body are known as the homeostatic mechanisms. Homeostasis also takes care of other demands. When you go out into the cold, and start to shiver, your homeostatic mechanisms are trying to warm you up. This is called *adaptation*: you are adapting to the cold.

When a cut is healing, the area will be red and inflamed. Inflammation is a sign that the homeostatic repair process is going on. This process of inflammation is necessary for recovery and tissue repair. Inflammation is a sign that your defence systems are adapting to, and repairing, the injury.

When you have an infection, your temperature goes up. This is a sign that the immune system is fighting (adapting to) the infection. The symptom is not pleasant (few symptoms are), but for recovery to take place it is essential that the bacteria or virus is overwhelmed by the homeostatic defences of the body. An elevated temperature is a sign that your defence systems are adapting to the infection.

But when your homeostatic mechanisms have to adapt to a great many things at the same time, they may not always be able to cope. Adaptation systems may begin to break down (see Figure 6.1, page 123). For example, someone may not be getting enough essential vitamins and/or minerals in the diet, and/or not getting adequate exercise, and/or has picked up a viral infection which never seems to quite go away, and/or is not sleeping well, and/or is under work and/or emotional stress, and/or has a slight hormonal imbalance. Each of these 'problems' (stresses) may be relatively minor, and could probably be sorted out by taking appropriate actions such as eating more sensibly, exercising more, ensuring a better sleep pattern, doing something positive about the stress, getting advice and treatment for the hormonal and the viral problems, etc.

But if nothing is done, and these various adaptive demands (and others) continue, the body's defence and repair systems can become so overloaded that they begin to break down. And as this happens, more chronic symptoms start to appear.

And of course, whatever emotional stress load, whatever nutritional deficiencies and acquired toxicities, and whatever biomechanical stresses (poor posture, tense muscles, poor breathing habits) are added to this 'load', all are being coped with in the context of the unique genetic characteristics which each of us is born with. Some people will have inborn abilities to handle some of the 'stress' load more efficiently than others.

Responses to similar stress burdens will therefore not be the same from one person to another.

What is the solution? One of two things needs to be done:

1. There is a need to stop, or to reduce, doing the things that are causing the adaptive demands which are overloading the system.
2. There is also a need to provide help to the repair and support systems of the body, and so to allow them to handle the adaptive load more efficiently.

If appropriate positive changes are made, the homeostatic repair systems may be able to start to work more efficiently again, to detoxify, fight infection, rebuild and repair, etc., and symptoms should gradually ease. In Chapter 6, the notes on homeostasis, as well as Figure 6.1, give a more in-depth picture of this vital subject. What is needed is that we do whatever we can to lighten the adaptive load, and as much as we can to help the body to handle its load better, so that health can be restored.

Some of the actions needed to help in recovery might involve providing nutritional, herbal or medical assistance, and/or there may be a need to learn to handle stress differently, using a variety of techniques. Specific action may be needed to deactivate painful trigger areas in the muscles, using bodywork or acupuncture or other techniques. The machinery of the body, the muscles and joints, may need to be toned and encouraged to work better, through better breathing and posture and exercise habits. Hormonal rebalancing may be necessary to restore equilibrium to the chemistry of the body, or whatever else may be needed to help to eliminate the adaptive demands that are loading the homeostatic systems.

When we come to consider a complex and debilitating condition such as fibromyalgia, it is possible to see that this is usually the result of a great many 'causes' interacting with the unique genetic makeup of the person involved. We should never lose sight of the self-repair aspect of the homeostasis story (as evidenced by the examples of the healing of cuts and colds discussed earlier). This process of self-repair is constant, but not always comfortable. So, keeping in mind the examples of inflammation and a high temperature, we need to accept that symptoms often represent evidence of healing in progress.

The questionnaires throughout this book will help to identify some of the changes which need to be made. And while a qualified and responsible health care professional may be required to guide one through the necessary dietary, herbal and other changes, in the end it is the person with the health problem who will need to make the choices and changes which can lead to a return to good health.

## Resources

On pages 262–265 there is a list of some of the many organizations in the USA that support people with fibromyalgia, chronic fatigue and associated conditions.

These organizations, and others not listed, provide useful information, support, articles, ideas, contacts, networks – usually for little or no cost.

# An Introduction to Fibromyalgia Syndrome (FMS)

Do you remember the last time you had flu? The aches, pains, stiffness, headache, lethargy, disturbed sleep, inability to concentrate, discomfort and sheer unpleasantness of it?

Imagine having flu all the time (but without the fever, and with the muscle pain as the strongest symptom) – for months or years – and you have an idea of what fibromyalgia syndrome (FMS) can be like.

Because fibromyalgia is a syndrome (a collection of symptoms and conditions), not everyone who has it has exactly the same symptoms. One person may have more pain than another, and some may be more exhausted than others, while many may feel more depressed or anxious than others.

Also, because doctors do not all agree, some people may be given a diagnosis of 'chronic fatigue syndrome', while others with very similar symptoms might be told they have fibromyalgia. Unfortunately, many people with exactly the same symptoms find it very difficult to get a diagnosis at all, and may be labelled as being 'neurotic' or 'depressed', when in fact their nervousness and depression are caused by the fact that they feel so physically awful.

Throughout this book, short questionnaires will be found. These are meant to help you to find answers, to know more about yourself and your condition. But they are *not* designed to help you to make a diagnosis. Only when *all* the different signs and symptoms are looked at together, by a qualified health care provider who has a full understanding of what they mean, can a diagnosis be made.

The questionnaires and the information in this book should be used to give you a deeper understanding of what may be happening to cause the symptoms you are feeling.

After each questionnaire, positive suggestions will be found which are aimed to encourage better health.

### The symptoms of fibromyalgia and the associated illnesses

The most common symptoms of fibromyalgia and conditions associated with it are:

- almost 100 per cent of sufferers have muscular pain, aching and/or stiffness (especially in the morning)
- almost 100 per cent have fatigue and badly disturbed sleep
- almost 100 per cent find that the symptoms are usually worse in cold or humid weather
- between 70 and 100 per cent (different studies have given different figures) suffer depression (though this is more likely to be a *result* of the muscular pain than be part of the *cause*)
- 34 to 73 per cent have Irritable Bowel Syndrome
- 44 to 56 per cent have severe headaches
- 30 to 50 per cent have Raynaud's phenomenon (in which the hands go white and cold)
- 24 per cent suffer from anxiety
- 18 per cent have dry eyes and/or mouth (Sicca syndrome)

- 12 per cent have osteoarthritis
- 7 per cent have rheumatoid arthritis
- an as yet unidentified number of people with fibromyalgia have had silicone breast implants; a newly identified silicone breast implant syndrome (SBIS) is now being defined
- between 3 and 6 per cent have substance (drugs and/or alcohol) abuse problems.

Other conditions extremely common among fibromyalgia sufferers include allergies, chronic rhinitis (an almost constantly runny nose), bruising easily, night cramps, restless leg syndrome, dizziness (sometimes caused by antidepressant medication taken to help the sleep problems experienced with fibromyalgia), sleep apnoea (when your breathing seems to stop while you are asleep), dry eyes and mouth, bruxism (teeth grinding), photophobia (extreme sensitivity to light), premenstrual syndrome, digestive disturbances, viral infections, Lyme disease (resulting from a tick bite), itchy skin – with or without a rash – loss of hair, sensitive bladder, mouth ulcers, generalized muscular stiffness, 'foggy' brain (difficulty in concentrating and poor short-term memory), dyslexia (the wrong words come out or what is read is not understood), panic attacks, phobias, mood swings, irritability and a feeling of the hands and feet being swollen without evidence of fluid retention. It has been noted, too, that commonly there is a history of injury – sometimes serious but often only minor – occurring within the year before the symptoms started.

## THE OFFICIAL DEFINITION OF FIBROMYALGIA

Many people suffer from generalized muscular aching and pain. However, this only *officially* becomes the medical condition labelled 'fibromyalgia syndrome' (FMS) when this aching muscle pain is accompanied by pain when pressure is applied to certain specific body areas.

The most commonly accepted definition (devised by the American College of Rheumatology in 1990) is that a person has fibromyalgia when they show the following.

- A history of widespread pain. Pain is considered 'widespread' when all of the following are present:
  - pain in the left side of the body
  - pain in the right side of the body
  - pain above the waist and pain below it
  - pain in the spine or the neck or front of the chest or thoracic spine or lower back.
- Pain in 11 out of 18 tender point sites when these are pressed with the fingers. There should be pain on pressure (around 4 kg/8 ¾ lb of pressure maximum) in no fewer than 11 of the following sites:
  - either side of the base of the skull, where the suboccipital muscles insert
  - either side of the side of the neck, between the fifth and seventh cervical vertebrae (technically described as between the 'anterior aspects of inter-tranverse spaces')
  - either side of the body on the midpoint of the muscle that runs from the neck to the shoulder (upper trapezius)
  - either side of the body on the origin of the muscle that runs along the upper border of the shoulder blade (the supraspinatus)
  - either side, on the upper surface of the rib, where the second rib meets the breastbone, and in the pectoral muscle on the outer aspect of either elbow, just below the main bone which can be felt (epicondyle)
  - in the large buttock muscles, either side, on the upper outer aspect, in the fold in front of the muscle (gluteus medius)

— just behind the large bump of either hip joint where the piriformis muscle inserts
— on either knee, in the fatty pad just above the inner aspect of the joint.

## Neutral points and other sites

When the specific sites just mentioned are being pressed, some healthcare professionals will also press 'neutral' or 'dummy' sites in order to see whether or not the person being assessed is suffering from a more widespread, generalized sensitivity that might be something other than fibromyalgia.

## When there are different pain reports under different circumstances

Experts say that there seems to be some variation in sensitivity of the tender points, due to age, sex and race. For example:

- Caucasians (white people of European stock) report more tender point sensitivity than do black races or Hispanics
- women report more tender points than men
- the number of tender sites reported increases with age, with the maximum noted around the age of 70, on average (F. Wolfe, 1985).

## How many points?

Disagreement exists over how many tender point sites are needed before you will be diagnosed as having fibromyalgia – whether 3, 7 or 11 areas of pain are needed for such a diagnosis. Over the years, the diagnostic rulings seem to have varied widely. At one time, 19 painful sites out of 75 tested were thought to be necessary, but this was later changed to 10 out of 25.

As we have seen, now, officially, 11 sites need to be found to be painful, out of 18 tested. However, international experts Drs Yunus, Simms and Rothschild state that they think only three are required, as long as putting pressure on these places produces the pain reported by the patient.

Alternatively, there could be sensitivity in almost all the points pressed, even the neutral points, which could lead (often wrongly) to the diagnosis that the pain is psychological in origin.

The difference between the current guidelines for diagnosing fibromyalgia and those for fibrositis (the old name for fibromyalgia) seems to lie in the number of tender points found. These were 5 or more for fibrositis, and are 11 or more for fibromyalgia, although, as we have just seen, there is not yet general agreement among experts on this last figure.

Thus, finding 11 tender points out of 18 sites tested by pressure can be enough to produce a diagnosis of fibromyalgia, as can 3 'referring' sites (trigger points) in patients who have chronic pain in all 'corners' of the body.

All patients diagnosed as having fibromyalgia have to meet some such criteria, either as set out by the official statement of the American College of Rheumatologists (see Figure 1.1) or as described by experts who take a different view. At least 75 per cent of people diagnosed as having chronic fatigue syndrome (CFS) will also meet these specific [fibromyalgia] criteria and can therefore also be diagnosed as having fibromyalgia syndrome (George Duna and William Wilke, 1993).

The similarities between fibromyalgia syndrome, chronic fatigue syndrome and Irritable Bowel Syndrome are listed in Table 1.1 (see the discussion below in this chapter and in Chapter 2 on the link between fibromyalgia and chronic fatigue syndrome).

In addition to these similar – indeed, identical – factors, *all* these conditions are also frequently characterized by pain, fatigue, headaches, disturbed sleep patterns, anxiety, depression, numbness and tingling in the arms, hands or feet, and bowel disturbances (diarrhoea and/or constipation on their own or alternating), which are all frequently affected by the weather, activity and stress, and there are usually many painful and sensitive areas to be found, on palpation,

**Figure 1.1** *These are the tender point sites as defined by the American College of Rheumatologists. Of the 18 points (9 sites each side of the body), at least 11 must be reported to be painful on mild pressure to allow an 'official' diagnosis of fibromyalgia to be made.*

in sufferers of all of them. Irritable bowel problems will usually be associated with areas in the abdomen that are painful when pressed.

In 1992, a 'Consensus Document on Fibromyalgia' was produced at the Second World Congress on Myofascial Pain and Fibromyalgia in Copenhagen (Consensus Document, 1992). This declaration accepted the American College of Rheumatologists' definition of FMS and added a number of symptoms to that definition (apart from widespread pain and multiple tender points) including persistent fatigue, generalized morning stiffness and non-refreshing sleep, headache, irritable bladder, dysmenorrhoea, extreme sensitivity to cold, restless legs, odd patterns of numbness and tingling, intolerance to exercise and others.

**Table 1.1** The similarities between fibromyalgia, chronic fatigue syndrome, and irritable bowel syndrome

|  | Fibromyalgia | Irritable bowel | Chronic fatigue |
| --- | --- | --- | --- |
| **Age** | Young adult | Young adult | Young adult |
| Primary sex | Female | Female | Female |
| Prevalence | Common | Common | Common |
| Cause | Not known | Not known | Not known |
| Chronic | Yes | Yes | Yes |
| Lab. studies | Normal | Normal | Normal |
| Pathological findings | None | None | None |
| Disabling | Yes | Yes | Yes |

The data in this table derives from S. Block, 'Fibromyalgia and the rheumatisms' *Controversies in Clinical Rheumatology*, 19 (1) p. 68, 1993: M. Yunus, 'Fibromyalgia and other functional syndromes', *Journal of Rheumatology*, 16 (sup. 19) (69), 1989, and D. Goldenberg, 'Fibromyalgia and its relationship to chronic fatigue syndrome, viral illness and immune abnormalities, *Journal of Rheumatology*, 16 (sup. 19) (92), 1989.

This declaration recognized that people with FMS may at times present with fewer than 11 painful points. In such a case a diagnosis of 'possible FMS' is appropriate, with a follow-up assessment suggested to reassess the condition.

## CHILDREN WITH FIBROMYALGIA
Many children are now being diagnosed as having fibromyalgia. It often starts with flu-like symptoms and then becomes chronic, with sleep disturbance as a major feature. Some children also display attention deficit disorder (ADD) symptoms, which are fatigue, school and behaviour problems and, commonly, a tendency to allergies. Some fibromyalgia experts also find that such children frequently have very loose (hypermobile) joints (see pages 41, 84 and 212).

## How many people are affected by fibromyalgia?

Muscular pain that goes on for months or years is now common, often causing sufficient disability to prevent people from working or functioning normally. In fact, fibromyalgia is now the most common disorder seen by rheumatologists after osteoarthritis and rheumatoid arthritis.

Dr. Don Goldenberg, Chief of Rheumatology at Newton-Wellesley Hospital and Professor of Medicine at Tufts University School of Medicine, estimates that there are between 3 and 6 million Americans affected by fibromyalgia, mainly between the ages of 26 and 35, and with the vast majority being women (86 per cent females against 14 per cent males according to many surveys).

Based on population size and surveys, we can therefore estimate that between 750 thousand and 1.5 million people in Britain also have fibromyalgia.

According to leading medical experts, in total it is estimated by Professor Bruce Rothschild of Northeast Ohio Universities College of Medicine, that nearly 25 per cent of patients seen at rheumatology clinics are actually suffering from fibromyalgia (1991).

A Norwegian study of nearly 250 young women with chronic musculoskeletal pain (aged 20 to 49) found that 10 per cent of them fully met the strict criteria for the diagnosis of fibromyalgia, while many more partly met them.

## How disabling is fibromyalgia?

Out of 394 patients, 100 (that is, 25.3 per cent) with fibromyalgia (all female), and 12 out of 44 males (27 per cent), were shown in a survey (presented to the 1994 American College of Rheumatology meeting by Don Goldenberg, MD) to be sufficiently badly affected by the condition as to be unable to work; they were, effectively, disabled (1993).

Almost all the others surveyed claimed that their fibromyalgia affected their job performance very badly. This survey found that those who were disabled by their fibromyalgia remained in great pain long after they'd received their disability benefits, which shows that stopping work brought them little or no relief.

In Canada, the insurance company London Life reported in 1989 that it was issuing monthly long-term disability payments to over 630 people who had been diagnosed as having fibromyalgia, which involved a total of around a million dollars a month.

## Clearing up the confusion about names and conditions

Just as 'fibrositis' has become 'fibromyalgia', 'chronic fatigue syndrome' has now replaced the terms 'chronic mononucleosis' and 'chronic Epstein-Barr syndrome' of the recent past, and those of 'neurasthenia' and 'nervous exhaustion' used in Victorian times.

There is still disagreement among experts as to whether chronic fatigue syndrome is the same as myalgic encephalomyelitis (ME, known in the USA as post-viral fatigue, PVFS) or not, and it seems likely that this argument will run for some time. In this book, wherever the chronic fatigue is not related to known disease processes, such as diabetes or clinical depression, or simply over-tiredness as a result of natural causes (such as overwork), we will refer to the two names together: chronic fatigue syndrome (ME).

Some doctors insist that the psychological aspects of these conditions are the most important cause, and so use the terms 'masked depression' and 'somatoform disorder' to describe such conditions. This is strongly resented by those afflicted by chronic fatigue syndrome (ME) or fibromyalgia, who see the psychological and emotional symptoms as being the result of their fatigue, pain and general ill-health, not the causes.

ARE CHRONIC FATIGUE SYNDROME (ME) AND FIBROMYALGIA THE SAME?
Fibromyalgia syndrome and chronic fatigue syndrome (ME) often seem to begin after an infection or a severe shock (physical or emotional), and the symptoms are very similar. The only obvious difference seems to be that, for some people, the fatigue

---

element dominates, while for others the muscular pain is their worst symptom.

In other words, for many people 'chronic fatigue syndrome' and 'fibromyalgia syndrome' are interchangeable terms, although there are certain symptoms (fever and swollen glands, for example) that are found in a higher percentage of chronic fatigue syndrome (ME) patients than those with fibromyalgia. The term chronic fatigue syndrome (ME) will be used together with fibromyalgia throughout this book to indicate that this large body of people has symptoms that it is widely acknowledged are often identical to those of fibromyalgia.

In 1988, Dr. Harvey Moldofsky tested chronic fatigue syndrome (ME) patients as well as fibromyalgia patients whose symptoms started after a flu-like illness (infection), and those whose symptoms started in other ways. He found that the electrical brain wave patterns (EEG brain anomalies), tender points, pain and fatigue were identical in all these groups (1993).

In 1993 Don Goldenberg, MD, compared 50 patients diagnosed as having fibromyalgia with 50 patients diagnosed with chronic fatigue syndrome (ME). He found that symptoms of a sore throat (54 per cent), rash (47 per cent), chronic cough (40 per cent), swollen lymph glands (33 per cent) and recurrent low-grade fever (28 per cent) were virtually the same in both groups. As these symptoms are common among chronic fatigue syndrome (ME) patients, it seemed likely to him that the diagnosis can often be interchangeable.

## FIBROMYALGIA AND MYOFASCIAL PAIN SYNDROME

There have also been debates among experts as to whether or not fibromyalgia is or is not the same as another painful muscle condition – myofascial pain syndrome. Some believe it is, and others are quite sure it is not (see also Chapter 4).

Yet other experts continue to use terms such as 'muscular rheumatism' or any of literally dozens of other similar words and terms to describe what is, essentially, exactly the same condition.

## WHAT'S IN A NAME?

Such arguments may not seem important, but they are a key factor in the lack of progress in addressing this widespread problem. As long as there remains no general agreement as to what name to give to a condition, there tends to be no concerted focus on research or on understanding what is going on. For years, the sometimes violent verbal debate as to whether or not ME was 'real' – was it 'all in the mind' or a real physical problem? – focused attention away from the profound suffering involved and prevented the real and dramatic progress via research that has since shown us so much of what is really going on in the brains and bodies of those afflicted.

It was only when researchers started taking the condition seriously – after the Centers for Disease Control labelled it 'chronic fatigue syndrome' and after a concerted campaign by sufferers for action – that scientists began to obtain research grants and clinicians could begin to look at treatment protocols without feeling that they were dealing with a mirage.

An example of why the naming of a condition matters can be seen when you look at the word 'fibrositis' (the previously used name for fibromyalgia, which means 'muscle pain').

When a word ends in 'itis' in medicine, it signifies that an inflammatory process is involved. However, no evidence has ever been produced that the muscular aches and pains which are among the main symptoms of fibrositis and/or fibromyalgia have much to do with inflammation.

It is not surprising, therefore, that anti-inflammatory drugs have no effect on the condition and, because of this, many doctors assumed that the condition itself was a fiction – that there was no such thing as fibrositis and that the symptoms complained of were unimportant or imaginary.

By changing its name to fibromyalgia syndrome, the inflammation element was removed from its name and, because the word 'syndrome' is part of its full name, this tells the doctor that there is more to the condition than just muscular pain.

The whole condition suddenly became more believable, and with this perception came the possibility of researching into it to acquire a wider understanding of the processes involved. Indeed, the change in name from fibrositis to fibromyalgia syndrome was accompanied by a sudden rash of research and review articles on it in the medical journals – there were only a few in 1985, but around 100 in 1990, and thousands today, although many still confuse the names used to describe the condition (Joseph Kalik, 1989).

It is true that none of these debates about what to call a disorder (of which we will hear more in Chapter 4) alters the unpleasant symptoms being experienced by hundreds of thousands of people one tiny bit, but it can help to explain why so much confusion exists among doctors and other healthcare professionals. Also, when the experts themselves have differing views, it is not surprising that there is no clearly defined procedure for those trying to help the person in pain.

## PATIENT POWER

Just as with chronic fatigue, it has been activists suffering or recovering from the condition who have helped most in clarifying just what is going on and bringing the most sensible information as to the needs of those suffering to the attention of the public, the media and the healing professions. Organizations such as ME Action in the UK and the Fibromyalgia Network in the USA are to be commended for the consistently professional and dedicated manner in which they have activated authorities and supported those affected.

### What should make you suspect that you might have fibromyalgia?

If you have chronic muscular pain (that is, you have been experiencing it for at least three months), affecting most areas of the body, and if a number of the particular sites listed by the American College of Rheumatologists (Don Goldenberg, 1993) feel painful when subjected to moderate pressure, even if there are no additional associated symptoms (such as sleep and bowel disturbances or fatigue) and whether or not the symptoms are affected by climatic factors, you may have fibromyalgia.

What you need to know next is what is actually happening to the body to produce the painful muscular (and other) symptoms, and then what can be done to help you.

In the coming chapters we will examine conditions that can be confused with fibromyalgia as well as some other health problems which seem to be associated with it. In these discussions we will learn of some of the most recent research findings, which will help to explain the way science is gradually coming to understand the processes involved.

# 2

# The Conditions and Symptoms Associated with Fibromyalgia

Fibromyalgia, as its full name tells us, is a syndrome. This means that it consists of far more than just the one main symptom, muscular pain – awful as this can be. (Note: The abbreviation 'FMS' is often used for fibromyalgia, 'CFS' for chronic fatigue syndrome, with 'ME' added to take account of the British name for the condition Myalgic Encephalomyelitis.)

In this chapter we will survey the most common and important of the associated conditions. You will find out, too, how they will be treated by your doctor, as well as ways of helping to treat yourself.

One of the most interesting lists of symptoms associated with fibromyalgia and chronic fatigue syndrome (ME) was that given to a conference on the subject in 1990 by Carol Jessop, MD, a leading physician from San Francisco. The number of patients with FMS or CFS/ME she has seen and studied (over a thousand) makes this a comprehensive selection of associated symptoms, and what is even more impressive is that many of her patients are referred to her by other physicians, which means that the diagnosis is more likely to be accurate because both she and the referring doctor have agreed that these people are suffering from fibromyalgia or chronic fatigue syndrome (ME).

## What the patients reported

The list of symptoms reported by Dr. Jessop's patients is as follows:

| | |
|---|---|
| chronic fatigue | 100 per cent |
| cold extremities | 100 per cent |
| impaired memory | 100 per cent |
| frequent urination | 95 per cent |
| depression | 94 per cent |
| sleep disorder | 94 per cent |
| balance problems | 89 per cent |
| muscle twitching | 80 per cent |
| dry mouth | 68 per cent |
| muscle aches | 68 per cent |
| headaches | 68 per cent |
| sore throat | 20 per cent |

Dr. Jessop stated that the symptom of depression was a 'reactive depression' not a 'clinical depression', and that only 8 per cent of her depressed patients had required prior medical attention for their depression before the symptoms of their chronic fatigue syndrome or fibromyalgia emerged.

## WHAT DR. JESSOP FOUND WHEN TESTING HER PATIENTS

Dr. Jessop also reported the following objective signs and findings among her 1,324 patients (their average age was 39; 75 per cent of them were female):

| | |
|---|---|
| tender neck muscles | 91 per cent |
| yeast infections (tongue or mouth) | 87 per cent |
| low blood pressure | 86 per cent |
| fibromyalgia tender spots | 86 per cent |
| white spots on nails | 85 per cent |

| | |
|---|---|
| abdominal tenderness | 80 per cent |
| subnormal temperature | 65 per cent |
| tender thyroid | 40 per cent |
| normal temperature | 25 per cent |
| swollen lymph nodes | 18 per cent |
| raised temperature | 10 per cent |

The symptom of a subnormal temperature possibly indicates an underactive thyroid. Later in this chapter the importance of the thyroid gland in fibromyalgia will become clearer. White flecks on the nails can sometimes be a sign of a zinc deficiency.

Of the 880 patients specifically tested, 82 per cent had yeast present in their stool samples. Also, 30 per cent of them were shown to have parasites in these samples. Yeast overgrowth is a major feature of some people's fibromyalgia and/or chronic fatigue. There is discussion of this possible connection later in this chapter.

### Deficiencies and CFS(ME)/FMS

To discover whether people are deficient in particular nutrients, tests called 'loading tests' are carried out. A known amount of the nutrient is taken (in this case zinc or magnesium) and then urine samples are tested to see what levels of the supplement find their way into the urine. The results of the urine tests and blood tests showed that low zinc and magnesium levels in fibromyalgia and chronic fatigue patients are common. Dr. Jessop believes that the analysis of sweat is a more accurate way of testing for zinc (a patch is worn on the arm for an hour and then tested to see the zinc levels in the sweat), but that it is not easy to carry out such a test in a normal office environment.

### PRIOR SYMPTOMS

Dr. Jessop stated that her patients had said that they had experienced a number of symptoms well before the onset of their chronic fatigue syndrome (ME) or fibromyalgia symptoms. For example:

| | |
|---|---|
| premenstrual symptoms | 90 per cent |
| irritable bowel symptoms | 89 per cent |
| recurrent childhood ear, nose and throat infections | 89 per cent |
| 'constant gas' or bloating | 80 per cent |
| endometriosis | 65 per cent |
| constipation | 58 per cent |
| heartburn | 40 per cent |
| recurrent sinusitis | 40 per cent |
| recurrent bronchitis | 30 per cent |
| dysmenorrhoea (painful or difficult periods) | 30 per cent |
| generalized anxiety disorders | 22 per cent |
| recurrent bladder infections | 20 per cent |
| sleep problems | 1 per cent |

It is worth noting just how many of these people had suffered from infections before they developed their chronic pain or fatigue symptoms. Most of the infections were almost certainly treated with course after course of antibiotics – the significance of this will become clear later in this chapter when we look at the 'yeast connection' and digestive distress.

### Further evidence of associated symptoms

Dr. Jessop is not the only researcher into the number and type of associated conditions and fibromyalgia.

Professor Danial Clauw has compared the symptoms of FMS patients (thought to be 2 per cent of the population) with those found in the rest (the other 98 per cent) of the population (or, where appropriate – for example with dysmenorrhoea – with the general female population).

Dr. Clauw's list of conditions are in alphabetical order – not in any order of importance (D. Clauw, 1995).

| Name | % in CFS/FMS | % general population |
| --- | --- | --- |
| chronic headache | 50% | 5% |
| dysmenorrhoea | 60% | 15% |
| Endometriosis | 15% | 2% |
| interstitial cystitis | 25% | under 1% |
| irritable bladder/urethral pain | 15% | under 1% |
| Irritable Bowel Syndrome | 60% | 10% |
| mitral valve prolapse | 75% | 15% |
| multiple chemical sensitivities | 40% | 5% |
| Restless Legs Syndrome | 30% | 2% |
| Temperomandibular Joint Syndrome | 25% | 5% |

Some of the really significant differences between what people who have CFS (ME)/FMS suffer from compared with those who do not can be seen to relate to bowel, bladder and menstrual problems, which agrees well with what Dr. Jessop's patients experienced before the onset of their conditions. This should alert people with such problems (irritable bowel or bladder for example) who do not have CFS(ME)/FMS, that they really should take action to try to get these conditions under control, as they seem to predispose towards more chronic ill-health. Advice will be found in this and later chapters (particularly Chapters 6 and 7) to guide you towards suitable strategies.

## FIBROMYALGIA NETWORK SURVEY EVIDENCE
In October 1997, the newsletter of the Fibromyalgia Network published information compiled from the more than 6,000 responses they had received to a survey questionnaire (Fibromyalgia Network Newsletter, 1997).

- 6,240 patients responded
- 97 per cent of these respondents had a diagnosis of FMS; 28 per cent had a diagnosis of CFS (with an overlap of a

double diagnosis in about a quarter of the respondents)
- average age was 52.6
- 95 per cent were female
- duration of illness averaged 12.2 years
- 7.2 years on average had passed before a diagnosis was made

Those patients with an FMS diagnosis reported the following associated symptoms:

| | |
|---|---|
| IBS or irritable bladder | 64 per cent |
| headaches | 59 per cent |
| chemical sensitivities | 26 per cent |
| osteoarthritis | 20 per cent |
| thyroid disease | 19 per cent |

When asked whether they could identify events which had 'triggered' their condition, 59 per cent indicated they could identify the trigger. The following were listed:

| | |
|---|---|
| physical injury | 39 per cent (of the 59 per cent who could identify a trigger) |
| major emotional shock such as bereavement | 27 per cent |
| infection | 15 per cent |
| surgery | 9 per cent |
| exposure to chemical agent or drug | 5 per cent |

The physical injury answer will be seen to have a particular relevance when we examine the link between FMS and whiplash injury in Chapter 4.

Asked about improvement or lack of it since their diagnosis, those with FMS offered these responses:

- 0.2 per cent had fully recovered
- 31 per cent had improved

- 20 per cent were unchanged
- 40 per cent were worse
- 9 per cent had become disabled

Newer methods of treatment – in particular, combinations of appropriate therapeutic interventions together with self-help measures, and specifically the use (where appropriate) of measures to correct thyroid imbalances – offer greater hope of recovery than these figures suggest. These measures will be outlined in later sections of this book.

The associated symptoms reported by the FMS responders (97 per cent of the survey) were:

| | |
|---|---|
| memory and concentration difficulties | 86 per cent |
| major discomfort following exertion | 89 per cent |
| waking tired in the morning | 89 per cent |
| unable to work because of FMS | 40 per cent |
| percentage of time spent in pain | 76 per cent |
| percentage of body in pain | 71 per cent |

When asked which health care disciplines were the most helpful and knowledgeable regarding their condition, the responses were as follows. The response findings are listed in descending order of patient satisfaction, that is, the first – rheumatologists – were most appreciated, and family physicians least appreciated in this survey. The percentage of the people responding to the questionnaire who were attending each discipline is placed in brackets.

1 rheumatologists (51 per cent)
2 physical medicine and rehabilitation specialists (13 per cent)
3 neurologists (10 per cent)
4 chiropractors (6 per cent)
5 internists (27 per cent)
6 family physicians (46 per cent)

When asked what was the most helpful on a scale of 1 to 10 (with 10 being the most helpful), the responses were:

drug and non-drug therapies                4.8 out of 10
educational material rated                 7.4 out of 10

Many research studies show that when people learn about their condition and begin to understand what may be happening to (and in) their own body, this is usually a great help. Anxiety grows when symptoms seem to be appearing for no reason, when functions seem to be vanishing, when it is not easy to think straight or to do things which were normal until recently – and when there is no explanation for what's going on.

Information and understanding are a great part of the battle to get well again.

### Allergies and chemical sensitivity/toxicity

This is surprisingly common in people with fibromyalgia – far more so than in people who do not have FMS/CFS (ME).

Put simply, people with allergies are more likely to develop fibromyalgia, and people with fibromyalgia are more likely than not to have allergies.

In a study at East Carolina University School of Medicine in 1992, involving approximately 50 people with hay fever or perennial allergic rhinitis (chronic runny nose), it was found that around half those tested fitted the criteria for fibromyalgia set by the American College of Rheumatology (Cleveland, 1992).

As between 2 and 5 per cent of the general population have fibromyalgia, the fact that 49 per cent of sufferers in the study had allergies points to there being a link between these two conditions.

A study in Seattle compared three groups of patients referred to a university-based clinic; these patients already had a diagnosis of either chronic fatigue syndrome (CFS), fibromyalgia syndrome (FMS) or multiple chemical sensitivities (MCS).What emerged was a picture of three conditions which were frequently difficult to distinguish from each other.

Fully 70 per cent of the patients with an FMS diagnosis, and 30 per cent of those with multiple chemical sensitivities, met all the criteria for chronic fatigue syndrome.

The researchers' conclusion was that it was difficult to clearly distinguish patients with CFS, FMS and MCS. Symptoms typical of each disorder are common in the other two conditions (D. Buchwald, 1994).

Turkish research evaluated the frequency of major symptoms in a group of over 30 patients with a diagnosis of 'primary fibromyalgia' compared people without FMS, and found that those with fibromyalgia had far more evidence of allergy than the people they were compared with (T. Tuncer, 1997).

Dr. Anne Macintyre, medical adviser to M.E. Action, an active patient support group for patients with chronic fatigue conditions in the UK, supports an 'immune dysfunction' model as the underlying mechanism for CFS(ME)/FMS. She states, 'The immune dysfunction may be associated with increased sensitivities to chemicals and/or foods, which can cause further symptoms such as joint pain, asthma, headache and IBS.' (A. Macintyre, 1993).

According to the Fibromyalgia Network Newsletter (October 1993), the official publication of fibromyalgia/chronic fatigue syndrome support groups in the USA, the foods that most commonly cause problems for many people with fibromyalgia or chronic fatigue syndrome (ME) are wheat and dairy products, sugar, caffeine, aspartame, alcohol and chocolate. Exclusion and rotation diets which can help to overcome these kinds of allergies are explained in Chapter 6.

THE CHEMICAL SENSITIVITY LINK

Chemical sensitivities or allergies are also common in people with fibromyalgia; it is thought by many experts that a percentage of people with this syndrome or chronic fatigue syndrome (ME) have probably been affected by toxic contamination, and that this is a major cause of their conditions. Such contamination is not always related to industrial settings.

According to Professor Gunnar Hauser, MD, of UCLA, 'Toxic exposure doesn't always occur in factories. There are many chemicals in our everyday environment (as well as those acquired from medical and social drug usage) that can lead to serious health problems, including household cleaners, new carpets, perfumes and certain types of paints.'

All the symptoms associated with fibromyalgia and chronic fatigue syndrome (ME) can result from such exposure.

When Dr. Hauser (Fibromyalgia Network Newsletters, 1993, 1994) sent 60 chemically-sensitive patients for brain scan evaluations, the same patterns that are found in fibromyalgia and chronic fatigue syndrome (ME) patients were discovered – a reduction of blood flow to and through specific parts of the brain dealing with memory and concentration, as well as pain-regulating functions (the caudate nuclei region, which has links with the limbic system). The limbic system works like a computer, controlling many functions – indeed, it is often called the 'emotional switchboard' of the body. This circulation disturbance to the brain may be one of the most important aspects of the cause of the symptoms of fibromyalgia (see Chapter 5).

A new twist to the chemical sensitivity and allergy link with fibromyalgia relates to what is now being called the Persian Gulf (or the 'Balkan War' or 'Kosovo') Syndrome, which is affecting thousands of people (troops and civilians alike) who were exposed to highly toxic compounds during these wars (see below). Reduced uranium used in the nose-cones of missiles is now considered a key element in producing many of these symptoms, particularly those which relate to disturbed thyroid function and immune system deregulation.

## YEASTS AND PARASITES AS CAUSES OF ALLERGIES

See also the discussion of this topic under the heading Candida (Yeast) Connections, page 34.

There can also be a connection between chemical sensitivity, allergies and chronic yeast (Candida) or parasite infections of the intestinal tract. More details of the yeast connection are found later in this chapter. Infestation of the bowels by yeast or parasites can result in damage to the delicate lining of the intestinal tract as well as reduced health and efficiency of the bowel flora (the 'friendly bacteria' that live in us and assist – among many other useful things – in detoxifying the body). This can lead to substances (food breakdown products, toxins and so on) being absorbed into the bloodstream from the gut, and these can trigger allergic symptoms (often including fatigue and muscle pain).

In this way, the allergies and irritable bowel conditions can be seen as two links in a chain of events in which fatigue (a common side-effect of allergies) and muscle pain can also occur.

Fortunately there exist safe ways of helping to heal the intestinal lining, as well as proven detoxification methods to overcome such problems. These are described in Chapter 6.

### Allergy questionnaire ?

The following questionnaire will help you to identify 'allergy' and 'sensitivity/intolerance' as possible factors in your health condition. The difference between something that happens sometimes, rather than always being a symptom, is that something which happens all the time usually relates to an ongoing process, such as toxicity; something that happens once or twice a day or several times a week probably relates to exposure to something in the environment, something you are periodically in contact with or which you sometimes eat or drink or inhale.

Many of the signs that there might be an allergy as part of the cause of your condition can occur for other reasons than allergy, but if more than five of the following questions are answered with a 'YES' then there is a good chance that allergy/sensitivity/ intolerance is a factor, and that the detoxification and other strategies outlined in Chapter 6 should help to reduce this.

| | | Yes | sometimes (more than once a week) | No |
|---|---|---|---|---|
| 1 | Is your nose stuffed up/runny? | | | |
| 2 | Do you have dark circles under your eyes? | | | |
| 3 | Do you get sudden feelings of weariness? | | | |
| 4 | Do your eyes water for no obvious reason? | | | |
| 5 | Do you have sudden mood swings? | | | |
| 6 | Do you suddenly lose concentration? | | | |
| 7 | Do you have food cravings? | | | |
| 8 | Do you get headaches for no obvious reason? | | | |
| 9 | Do you get sudden feelings of rapid heart rate? | | | |
| 10 | Do you get skin rashes for no obvious reason? | | | |
| 11 | Do pains suddenly get worse for no obvious reason? | | | |
| 12 | Do you have digestive and/or bowel problems for no obvious reason? | | | |

If you answered YES more than five times, especially to one or more of the first three questions, then consider that allergy or intolerance may be part of the cause of your health problems. Refer to the notes in Chapter 6 in particular on this subject.

The 'pulse test' and other strategies to help confirm the possibility of allergy are also to be found in Chapter 6.

## Anxiety and/or hyperventilation and fibromyalgia

It is important to distinguish between those people with fibromyalgia who are also suffering from various psychological disturbances (anxiety, depression and so on), and those who feel emotional and/or depressed because of their constant pain, disturbed sleep and fatigue. Sadly, some doctors still blame the whole syndrome of muscle pain, fatigue, sleep disorder, etc. on the psychological status of sufferers rather than understanding that they feel this way as a result of these nagging and disabling symptoms.

A pioneer researcher into fibromyalgia is Dr. Muhammad Yunus, a clinician who has stated that 'The central features of FMS are independent of the psychological status and are more likely related to (i.e., resulting from) the FMS itself – although pain severity may be influenced by psychological factors.'

Dr. Yunus (1989) investigated the links between anxiety, stress and sleep disorders and found that, while these factors influence the intensity of the symptoms in FMS, they are not the cause. However, he suggests that psychological factors should never be ignored in people with fibromyalgia, because they can be aggravating factors where pain is concerned – just as they can in any other painful condition such as rheumatoid arthritis or some forms of cancer.

In an attempt to redirect the focus of physicians correctly, Dr. Yunus speaks of the 'disturbed physician syndrome' (DPS). He says, 'DPS (that is, doctors treating people with FMS) people are troubled because of their preoccupations that FMS patients are psychologically disturbed. It is not the FMS patients who are disturbed, it is the physicians who are psychologically disturbed because they ignore the data and whatever data there is they manipulate to say what they want.'

Anxiety can stem from being permanently in pain, chronically tired and suffering from a list of other associated symptoms. It can also act as an aggravating factor and, therefore, deserves consideration in any treatment plan.

## THE LINK BETWEEN FIBROMYALGIA AND BREATHING PROBLEMS

Dr. Mark Pellegrino of Ohio State University has studied fibromyalgia and its link with chest pain (Fibromyalgia Network Newsletters, 1993, 1994). He notes that 'FMS patients are more prone to getting anxiety or panic attacks, especially when placed in a stressful situation.'

As we will see, breathing irregularities often have a connection with the symptoms of anxiety. Hyperventilation and anxiety also have an intimate link with a lack of ability to cope with stress. At their simplest, the connections can look as follows:

- a person responds to a stressful situation by breathing shallowly, using the upper chest and not the diaphragm
- this breathing pattern becomes a habit, so that it continues when the stress is not present (even when sleeping), although it tends to be much more obvious when they are stressed
- with such a pattern of breathing, the accessory breathing muscles (these are the muscles connecting the neck and head with the upper ribs, which are normally active when we are puffing after running, for example) become overactive, tense and often develop painful local areas as a result of this overuse
- headaches due to the irritation of local nerve structures in these muscles and/or interference with circulation to and drainage from the head can occur – with possibly lightheadedness and dizziness prior to the headaches

- the overbreathing pattern leads to too much carbon dioxide being breathed out; this causes carbonic acid levels in the blood to be lowered, which then leads to the blood becoming too alkaline
- this alkalinity leads automatically to a feeling of apprehension or anxiety and to the abnormal breathing pattern becoming worse, and so panic attacks and even phobic behaviour are not uncommon following this
- the alkalinity also leads to nerve endings becoming increasingly sensitive, so that the individual is more likely to report 'pain', when previously 'discomfort' would have been how they would have described it
- when we are more alkaline, the levels of histamine (which is always circulating in the blood) rises and allergic reactions become more likely and stronger
- excessive alkalinity causes the smooth muscles around blood vessels to tighten, reducing the amount of blood which can get through to nourish muscles, the brain, etc. This is one of the reasons for lightheadedness, dizziness and 'brain-fog'
- inadequate oxygenation and the retention of acid wastes in overused muscles makes them become painful and stiff
- if the muscles being overused as a result of the inappropriate breathing pattern are mainly the postural, stabilizing muscles (the chest and neck muscles), they will, with the repetitive stress involved in the overbreathing, become short, tight and painful and will develop localized pain spots called trigger points (the most common sites for tender and trigger points lie in just these muscles of the neck, shoulder and chest!)
- the increased tension in these muscles adds a lot to feelings of fatigue as the muscles are constantly using energy in a non-productive way, even during sleep

- the poor breathing pattern leads to a restriction of the joints where the ribs attach to the spine, which, because they are not moving much due to the shallow breathing, are deprived of their normal, regular movements, leading to stiffness and discomfort there
- where the ribs attach to the breastbone (sternum) they are similarly restricted, leading to pain in this region
- a similar lack of movement of the diaphragm leads to the digestive organs missing out on the regular, rhythmic 'massage' they would normally receive as the diaphragm rises and falls
- shallow breathing prevents the useful pumping mechanism between the chest and the abdomen from taking place, which normally assists in returning blood from the legs and the rest of the lower body to the heart, so cold feet and legs could be a symptom of this
- the muscles between the ribs become tense and tight and there will be a likelihood of chest pain and a feeling of an inability to get a full and deep breath.

The end result of this breathing pattern is a stiff and painful neck and chest region, with associated sensitive and painful areas in the chest – back and front – headaches, dizziness, lightheadedness, fatigue (because of the inadequate oxygen supply to the body tissues and all the energy being wasted in keeping muscles constantly tense), a sense of anxiety, possible indigestion and poor circulation, along with a possible tendency to panic attacks and phobic behaviour.

Because this breathing pattern continues during sleep, nights are likely to be disturbed, too.

This scenario is not meant to suggest that fibromyalgia is *always* caused by a tendency towards shallow overbreathing, but it can certainly be seen to have links with many of the common symptoms of the syndrome, and therefore is something which should be attended to. Breathing retraining and other treatments can be used to minimize problems of the waste of energy and the mechanical stress to the muscles and joints of the neck, shoulder and chest region in particular.

After some 15 years of treating fatigue problems and over 30 years of treating musculoskeletal pain problems, I can categorically state that I have seldom, if ever, failed to find at least some degree of breathing dysfunction in people with chronic fatigue syndrome (ME) or fibromyalgia. Sometimes it is a major element, sometimes only a part of the picture, but it is almost always involved to some significant degree. Suggestions and breathing exercises aimed at normalizing breathing are given in Chapter 6.

## Overbreathing (hyperventilation) questionnaire ?

By taking this questionnaire you should be able to get an idea of whether you have a tendency to overbreathe, which really means that the amount of oxygen ($O_2$) you breathe in, and the amount of carbon-dioxide ($CO_2$) you breathe out, are out of balance with your actual bodily needs. Breathing this way can aggravate nearly all the symptoms of FMS/CFS(ME) and is usually just a habit. Breathing retraining (see Chapter 6) can help to correct this.

1   When you stand in front of a mirror and breathe, do your shoulders rise towards your ears? If the answer is YES, you are activating the 'wrong' muscles and are probably an upper-chest breather and may have a tendency to hyperventilation.

2   Still standing in front of the mirror, put one flat hand just above your navel and the other flat hand on your upper chest, below your throat. Take a deep breath. Which hand moves first? Does the upper hand move upward towards your chin? If the hand on your chest moves first and it also moves towards your chin as you inhale, this is a sign of upper chest breathing, and you may have a hyperventilation tendency.

3   Breathe out, and hold your breath out. Time how long it is before you feel the need to take another breath. If it is less than 20 seconds, you have a low tolerance to $CO_2$ and probably overbreathe. If it is less than 10 seconds you are either asthmatic or are in need of breathing retraining as a priority.

4   Do you sometimes feel lightheaded or dizzy, for no obvious reason?

5   Do you sometimes feel numbness or tingling in your legs or arms/hands for no obvious reason?

6   Does your stomach become bloated for no obvious reason? (This can be because of too much 'air swallowing', which accompanies upper chest breathing and is reduced or stopped when breathing is corrected.)

7   Do you suffer from poor concentration, short-term memory lapses or 'brain-fog'?

8   Do you suffer from anxiety, panic attacks and/or phobias?

Your answers to questions 1, 2 and 3 suggest whether or not you have a tendency to hyperventilate. Answering YES to questions 4, 5, 6, 7 or 8 (especially 8) should confirm this.

**Brain changes**
See also Chapters 5 and 6 for more on this subject, but a brief mention is relevant here.

A number of researchers have uncovered major changes in the function of brain circulation as well as the biochemistry of the brain in chronic fatigue syndrome (ME) and fibromyalgia sufferers (the picture is virtually the same for all of them). The changes are that:

■   substance P, a chemical compound which increases the sensitivity of nerves to pain, has been found in raised levels in the cerebrospinal fluid of people with fibromyalgia

- levels of the neurotransmitter serotonin have been found to be lower in people with chronic fatigue syndrome (ME) and fibromyalgia.This has a profound influence on sleep patterns as well as on the intensity of pain, so the implications are of some importance to sufferers as well as to researchers, who can then try to find out why this imbalance occurs and what can be done to normalize it
- chronic fatigue syndrome (ME) patients have been scanned using positron emission tomography (PET) and the scans have shown that certain areas of the brain are underactive in their uptake of glucose, which is the energy supply for the brain (these findings could explain aspects of the 'foggy brain' syndrome)
- the rate of blood flow in the brain can be tested using single photon emission computerized tomography (SPECT) scanning. When chronic fatigue syndrome (ME) sufferers as well as healthy individuals were studied in this way, it was discovered that the affected sufferers had poorer circulation to important parts of the brain controlling both memory and the movement of body parts, including the muscles
- brain electrical activity mapping (BEAM) was used to test chronic fatigue syndrome (ME) and fibromyalgia sufferers with abnormalities in circulation to the brain. The researchers found that it was impossible, using this test, to distinguish between chronic fatigue syndrome (ME) and fibromyalgia sufferers, even if the fibromyalgia sufferers did not report difficulties with memory.

Various constitutional (non-specific) treatment methods described in later chapters can be used, such as hydrotherapy, massage and deep relaxation, as well as several herbal (see notes in Chapter 6 on *Ginkgo biloba*) and nutritional methods to help to create a more normal blood flow to and through the brain. Craniosacral treatment by a suitably qualified practitioner can also be helpful.

## Candida (yeast) connections

Dr. Carol Jessop reported (see page 16) that nearly 90 per cent of her patients with fibromyalgia (men and women) had yeast infections, and that the vast majority of these had records of recurrent antibiotic use – commonly for sinus, acne, prostate, urinary tract and chest infection problems. Of the women, 70 per cent with chronic fatigue syndrome or fibromyalgia had been on the contraceptive pill for three years or more, and 63 per cent reported having a craving for sugar.

The use of antibiotics and steroid medication (including the contraceptive pill) can lead to the spread in the intestinal tract and the body generally of yeasts which normally live in confined areas of the body, controlled by 'friendly' bacteria – these medications upset the normal balance. The main yeast engaged in such activity is *Candida albicans*, which is best known for causing thrush.

Candida is potentially dangerous because of its ability to turn from a simple yeast into an aggressive fungus that puts down 'rootlets' (rhizomes) into the mucous membranes of the intestinal tract, therefore permitting undesirable toxins to move from the gut into the bloodstream, with the strong possibility that allergic and toxic reactions will then take place. This so-called 'leaky gut syndrome' may help to account for the allergy symptoms suffered by many people who also have irritable bowels.

Among the many symptoms of yeast overgrowth, especially in people who have a sugar-rich diet (yeast thrives on sugar!), are various digestive problems (bloating, swings from diarrhoea to constipation and back), urinary tract infections, menstrual disturbances, fatigue, muscle aches, emotional disturbances, 'foggy' brain symptoms and skin problems. The frequency with which such symptoms are suffered by people with fibromyalgia is too obvious to ignore.

A medical history that includes antibiotic use in anything other than brief or few instances, a high-sugar diet and/or the use of steroid medication (including the contraceptive pill) are the chief factors predisposing someone to yeast overgrowth. Laboratory tests are commonly inconclusive in diagnosing Candida, although one of the most useful involves a sugar-loading test, which assesses blood alcohol levels before and after a sugar intake (yeast – and some bacteria – can turn sugar into alcohol rapidly in the intestines). More complicated tests may involve an analysis of the stool, as this can often show precisely which yeasts are present in the gut as well as other aspects of the environment of the intestines. A strategy for managing Candida is given in Chapter 6.

## Candida (yeast) overgrowth questionnaire **?**

The questions in these two lists (Questionnaire A is mainly about medications you may have taken, Questionnaire B about symptoms) are designed to give you an idea as to whether yeast might be a part of your problem. It is not possible from the answers you give to make a diagnosis, but a strong suggestion can be gained. In order to get a definitive diagnosis you need to consult a health care professional who is suitably trained and licensed to make such a diagnosis, and to advise you how best to handle the problem. Recovery from a serious yeast over growth can take 6 to 12 months of carefully applied dietary and other strategies – as described in Chapter 6.

### Questionnaire A

1   Have you ever had a course of antibiotics which lasted for eight weeks or more, or for shorter periods more than four times in one year?

2   Have you ever been treated for acne with antibiotics for more than one continuous month?

3   Have you ever been treated with steroid drugs such as cortisone, ACTH or Prednisone?

4   Have you ever been treated with immunosuppressive drugs?

5   Have you been pregnant more than once?

6   Have you taken the contraceptive pill for more than one continuous year?

## Questionnaire B

1   Do you have a history of persistent vaginitis, cystitis or prostatitis?

2   Have you a history of endometriosis?

3   Have you had oral or vaginal thrush within the past three years?

4   Have you currently fungal infections of the nails or skin (such as athlete's foot or ringworm)?

5   Have you been diagnosed as having 'chronic fatigue'?

6   When you are exposed to chemical fumes, perfumes or tobacco smoke, are you badly affected?

7   Are your symptoms worse after eating yeast-containing (or sugary) foods?

8   Do you crave sweet foods, bread or alcohol such as beer or wine?

9   Do you suffer from abdominal bloating *and* either constipation or diarrhea?

10  Are you subject to allergies?

If you answered one or more of the questions in Questionnaire A with YES, and two or more of the questions in Questionnaire B with YES, then there is a reasonable possibility that yeast overgrowth is a part of your current health problems. Details will be found in the Useful Publications and Addresses section at the end of this book regarding ways of obtaining a laboratory assessment which can confirm the suggestion which these questionnaires raise. (This section also gives suggested reading and details of support groups.)

Strategies for successfully getting yeast under control are given in Chapter 6.

## Chest pain
See under Anxiety and/or Hyperventilation and Fibromyalgia, above.

## Depression
The fact that signs of depression are noted in people with chronic fatigue syndrome (ME) and fibromyalgia should not be surprising – there can be few more depressing situations than being constantly tired, lethargic and in pain! This misery is made worse when there is a lack of understanding on the part of health care providers as to the hell the sufferer is enduring or how to help.

The diagnosis of depression as the *cause* of the condition is now discredited, as most depression related to fibromyalgia is a direct *reaction* to the condition (loss of health) and so it is not a clinical depression, which is an endogenous, or self-produced, condition, unlike reactive depression which is a response to 'something'. In this case the reaction is to the symptoms of the illness.

It is worth considering for a moment that 'depression' is a perfectly normal human response to certain circumstances, and not necessarily an 'illness'. The same can be said for 'anxiety', because if someone is not anxious when faced with major problems, they are unlikely to respond appropriately. It is only when anxiety is excessive or inappropriate that it becomes a problem. Similarly, when certain life-events (such as bereavement) take place, or when circumstances are really difficult, a degree of withdrawal and depression is a perfectly normal response to the situation. Depression and anxiety only become 'problems' when these symptoms exist without sufficient cause, and when they go on for longer than is appropriate.

In the case of someone with FMS/CFS (ME), where it sometimes feels as though the body is falling apart and the mind is not far behind, it would be strange indeed if the person did not feel anxious and to an extent depressed. This is why there is such an enormous amount of relief when the condition is understood and explained. At least there is then a chance of doing something positive about the condition. Unfortunately in modern society the word 'depression' has a negative connotation, and people feel embarrassed to have this perfectly reasonable label attached to how they feel in response to being so ill.

The fact that for some people antidepressant medication helps to restore sleep patterns to some degree of normality and therefore minimizes the symptoms of fibromyalgia should not be taken to indicate that depression causes the syndrome – it usually does not.

Low doses of antidepressant medication may be appropriate, as might nutritional interventions that help to balance serotonin levels, or herbal antidepressants such as St John's Wort, which has fewer side-effects than pharmaceutical antidepressants. If the pain and fatigue elements of FMS/CFS can be modified, depression usually fades away.

### Fatigue

The tiredness experienced in chronic fatigue syndrome (ME) and fibromyalgia is not a normal response to activity which soon passes. Indeed, the fatigue and muscular pain felt by people with fibromyalgia after even mild activity often gets worse for several days following the activity, despite rest. If someone is not getting enough rest or sleep, it is perfectly normal to feel tired. The sort of fatigue which occurs in CFS and FMS is unnatural, excessive and far beyond what we experience with normal 'tiredness', and it usually does not feel better for rest. People with FMS/CFS often wake up (even if they manage to sleep reasonably) feeling tired and washed out.

Chronic fatigue is a major symptom of fibromyalgia and it is certainly not easy to distinguish between people with chronic fatigue syndrome (ME) and fibromyalgia, except that in the former the fatigue element is probably more dominant than the pain symptoms, while people diagnosed as having fibromyalgia have muscular pain as their main symptom.

Both groups of patients frequently suffer sleep disturbances, both suffer fatigue and are affected by weather changes, and muscular pain is a common feature of both. Even the swollen glands, sore throats and low-grade fever experienced by many people with chronic fatigue syndrome (ME) are also reported by many fibromyalgia sufferers. The British name for severe chronic fatigue, myalgic encephalomyelitis (ME), indicates that there is a muscular component to this form of chronic fatigue (the word 'myalgia' stems from the Greek for muscle).

In most respects, treatment that helps people with chronic fatigue syndrome (ME) will also help people with fibromyalgia.

Probably the most important warning that can be given to anyone who is chronically fatigued with an ME or post-viral fatigue condition, whatever the degree of muscular involvement, is that a return to normal activity should be cautious and slow. A common error, as symptoms eventually come under control or improve, is to try to do too much too soon, often with the unfortunate result of a return of exhaustion.

The natural desire to return to full activity needs to be curbed so that gains can be built on and not destroyed by excessive activity before stamina and strength are restored.

The use of constitutional hydrotherapy methods, relaxation and (when appropriate) aerobic exercises, appropriate bodywork, a structured and balanced diet that takes into account both toxicity and allergy factors, as well as specific medical or herbal or homoeopathic or acupuncture interventions where appropriate, form a holistic approach to restoring energy and wellbeing. The exact form the programme of treatment will be individual to each person. Many of these ideas are explored in later chapters.

### Growth hormones
See under Sleep Problems, below.

### Headaches
These occur chronically in over half of the fibromyalgia patients who have been surveyed. Most are of the migraine type, (usually one-sided throbbing, accompanied by nausea and sensitivity to light and sound), or the tension-type headache (which is characterized by a sensation like a tight band around the head, the forehead or the sides of the head). Tension headaches are commonly linked with neck tension or stiffness, and may be caused by active trigger points in the neck muscles. (See Chapter 4 for more details of trigger points.)

Both forms of headache can be relieved by various types of medication, as well as by a variety of natural approaches including bodywork, dietary changes, relaxation methods, acupuncture, homoeopathy and herbal medicine. Each person requires specific help tailored to their own particular needs.

Migraines are frequently linked to allergies (alcohol, particularly red wine, and caffeine – coffee, cola drinks, etc. – are two common triggers). If there is any such link, the trigger needs to be identified and eliminated. Migraines may also be related to hormonal variations, and stress is a key feature in both forms of headache, so learning some strategies for coping with stress can be useful.

Dr. Thomas Romano studied 100 people diagnosed as having fibromyalgia who also suffered chronic headaches, using the latest SPECT scanning methods (Fibromyalgia Network Newsletters, 1993, 1994). Of these, 97 showed blood flow differences between the right and left hemispheres of the brain, which led him to conclude that the imbalance in circulation was responsible for the headaches.

The frequent reports of the benefits experienced as a result of cranial therapy (craniosacral or cranial osteopathic treatment) and other forms of bodywork by people with chronic fatigue syndrome (ME) or fibromyalgia could be because of the very specific influences these essentially gentle treatment methods produce on both circulation to, and drainage from, the head. See also the details of the influence on pain conditions of the small muscles at the base of the skull (such as rectus capitis posterior minor) which are discussed in Chapter 4.

### Heart problems and fibromyalgia – the mitral valve prolapse connection

Dr. Pellegrino has evaluated the presence in fibromyalgia patients of a tendency for one of the heart valves (the mitral valve) to bulge (known as mitral valve prolapse) during the heartbeat (Fibromyalgia Network Newsletters, 1993, 1994).

A surprising 75 per cent of the 50 fibromyalgia sufferers tested (three-quarters of whom were women) had this usually harmless defect.

The connection between fibromyalgia and mitral valve prolapse may relate to a genetic connective tissue abnormality which leads to a lack of 'tone'. Such people may also be loose in their joints ('double jointed'). Mitral valve prolapse is not a heart disease and seldom requires treatment.

### Hyperventilation

See under Anxiety and/or Hyperventilation and Fibromyalgia, above, particularly the Overbreathing (Hyperventilation) questionnaire on page 31.

### Irritable bowel syndrome

This condition has been shown in research to affect at least three quarters of fibromyalgia sufferers (fewer in some studies than others, but always a significant number; see Dr. Jessop's figures at the beginning of this chapter).

The range of symptoms of Irritable Bowel Syndrome include alternating diarrhoea and constipation, abdominal gas or bloating, nausea, just diarrhoea or just constipation.

An Irish study examined people who had been diagnosed as having Irritable Bowel Syndrome and found that 65 per cent of them could also be diagnosed as having fibromyalgia, so it is clear that the two conditions are closely associated (Fibromyalgia Network Newsletters, 1993, 1994). Complementary therapists usually check for possible yeast or bacterial overgrowth, or for the presence of parasites (such as *Giardia lamblia*) in the intestinal tract, and the treatments they offer for these are described in Chapter 6. Some self-help treatments are available, though usually expert advice is required to help normalize chronic yeast and/or parasite problems. Stress reduction is also usually useful.

### Numbness and tingling of the hands and/or feet

These commonly have a mechanical cause, involving a restriction in circulation or nerve supply due to tense muscles or joint restriction, which can affect areas such as between the collar-bone and ribs at the base of the side of the neck (the thoracic inlet). When muscles become tense or the ribs or collar-bone are restricted due to injury or postural or repetitive strains, it is not uncommon for the hands to become numb and to tingle, especially at night.

Manipulative and other bodywork methods can usually help with such problems.

As noted in the discussion of anxiety and hyperventilation, these symptoms are also a frequent result of the biochemical changes which overbreathing produces.

### Painful muscles and/or joints

See Chapter 4.

**Persian gulf syndrome (also known as 'Balkan War', or 'Kosovo' syndrome)**

See also under Allergies and Chemical Sensitivity/Toxicity, under the section entitled The Chemical Sensitivity Link.

Many thousands of veterans of recent wars in the Persian Gulf and the Balkans (former Yugoslavia) are now reporting a long list of symptoms – unexplained joint and muscle pain, fatigue, difficulty sleeping, memory and/or concentration problems, headaches, hair loss, chest pain, breathing problems, gastrointestinal problems, skin rashes, allergies to foods and odours . . . and so on. And a significant number are also developing fatal blood diseases and cancer.

Experts are on record as stating that, in many instances, what is being complained of has the same symptom characteristics as fibromyalgia.

What are the causes? Most participants in these wars received a number of immunizations against the usual diseases, but also ones against anthrax and botulinus toxin (in anticipation of biological warfare) as well as taking anti-nerve gas pills (pyridostigmine bromide). Vehicles were sprayed with chemical agent-resistant coatings, and areas surrounding the military operations were sprayed with pesticides. There was also the use of armour-piercing reduced uranium armaments. Numerous oil-well fires and atmospheric pollution was another feature, as well as diesel exhausts, solvents vaporized by intense heat, poor hygiene (despite best efforts) and extremes of stress.

In investigating the condition, experts note that there is a direct link between what is inhaled and the brain, as the brain has no protective shield against all these chemicals. Limbic dysfunction due to chemical overload (multiple chemical sensitivities) is therefore one possible explanation for the symptoms described above. These possibilities are discussed in a review article in the July 1994 issue of *Fibromyalgia Network*, as is the alternative diagnosis of post-traumatic stress disorder.

Detoxification treatment has been attempted at some Veterans Administration centres. This involves living in a very pure environment (using air purifiers in all living areas), taking part in stress-reduction programmes and endurance and exercise classes, along with detoxification through rotation and elimination diets. So far, conclusive results are not available, but this approach at least seems to be dealing with some aspects of the toxic overload imposed on the more than 30,000 individuals who have reported symptoms of Gulf War syndrome (many thousands are probably still in military service and statistics on these people are not available). The possible damage to the immune system caused by the cocktail of immunizations received (on top of everything else the immune system had to deal with) would seem to be far more difficult to correct. The tragic radiation effects following exposure to reduced uranium dust is not calculable, but has undoubtedly proved to be fatal in many instances. Radiation exposure almost always involves thyroid function, which is discussed later in this chapter.

## Premenstrual syndrome

Of Dr. Jessop's patients (see earlier in this chapter), 90 per cent had reported symptoms of premenstrual tension – most of them having these symptoms well before their fibromyalgia or chronic fatigue syndrome symptoms started. Nearly 65 per cent had symptoms of endometriosis as well.

Many of the symptoms associated with premenstrual syndrome (fatigue, bloating, muscular pains, sleep disturbance, headaches, anxiety, swelling in the extremities, depression, confusion, emotional instability and so on) are common to chronic fatigue syndrome (ME) and fibromyalgia, too. The fact that these symptoms are periodic and not constant is the distinguishing factor between premenstrual syndrome and these more chronic conditions. They do allow us to glimpse certain possible contributing elements in the maze of potential causes involved in chronic fatigue syndrome (ME) and fibromyalgia, though. Apart from these common symptoms, there are the widely co-existing yeast overgrowth problems that women suffering premenstrual syndrome exhibit, and we have Dr. G. Abramson's classic research which has shown a direct link between specific nutrient deficiencies and these symptoms – particularly magnesium (of which more on pages 64, 144, 244) and vitamin $B_6$, which is closely linked to the conversion of tryptophan (a protein fraction) to serotonin, which, as we have seen, is considered by many experts to be deficient in the brains of those with fibromyalgia.

Nutritional and herbal treatments for the different categories of premenstrual syndrome are described in Chapter 6.

### Raynaud's phenomenon

This is also known as cold-induced vasospasm. It has been observed in up to 40 per cent of fibromyalgia sufferers according to some studies. The symptoms are the toes or fingers going dead white, or blue, when even slightly cold.

There are specific biochemical changes involved in this condition, which can often be helped by various forms of medication, as well as by bodywork techniques, acupuncture and deep forms of relaxation induced by biofeedback or autogenic training techniques, in which the person learns to partially influence the flow of blood to the hands or feet.

There are often links to food allergies, and certain nutrient supplements have been shown to help relieve this problem. See Chapter 6 for nutritional guidelines.

### Sicca syndrome

The chief characteristics of this are dry eyes and mouth, which may also burn and itch. Sometimes the dry mouth symptoms relate to side-effects of antidepressant medication such as amitriptyline, or to various forms of painkilling medication.

The eye and mouth symptoms should not be confused with similar symptoms common in a rheumatic condition called Sjögren's syndrome (which also commonly involves dryness of the skin as well as nasal and vaginal passages).

A key researcher into fibromyalgia, Dr. Don Goldenberg, has found that around 18 per cent of people with fibromyalgia have Sicca syndrome, which is thought sometimes to be part of an autoimmune dysfunction (where the body's defence mechanisms seem to attack the body itself). In a number of other autoimmune conditions (for example ankylosing spondylitis/AK and rheumatoid arthritis/RA), research has shown a connection between particular bacterial overgrowth in the intestinal tract and the conditions (*Klebsiella* in AK, *Proteus* in RA). Similar 'gut connections' may well be part of the evolution of other autoimmune conditions as well, even though the particular organisms which are triggering the misguided defence response have not as yet been identified.

Other possible contributing causes of this distressing dryness can be ongoing yeast infections of the mouth or vagina (such as Candida, which is always overgrown in the intestines as well, when it is active in other parts of the body) or the side-effects of silicone implants that leak (see below).

A variety of medical aids are available that offer relief from the symptom of dryness, including artificial 'tears' and water-based lubricants, and attention should always be paid to the health of the digestive tract.

## Silicone breast implant syndrome

Silicone implants leak and sometimes burst (apparently 70 per cent rupture by the time they have been in the body for 10 years), and the results of this range from autoimmune diseases such as lupus to scleroderma and possibly rheumatoid arthritis. The most common symptoms of silicone breast implant syndrome are pain (painful joints such as the shoulder), which occurs in almost all of those diagnosed, muscle pain (80 per cent), neurological problems (77 per cent), flu-like sensations (78 per cent), fatigue (78 per cent), dry eyes and mouth (60 per cent), Raynaud's phenomenon (48 per cent), and sleep disorders and chest pain mimicking a heart attack

(Fibromyalgia Network Newsletters, 1993, 1994, P. Baldry, 1993, Robert Cantu and Alan Grodin, 1992, Don Goldenberg, 1993, Beth Ediger, 1991). In different studies of people with silicone implants, fibromyalgia symptoms were found in between 25 and 50 per cent of patients.

Detoxification methods such as those mentioned under Allergies and Chemical Sensitivity/Toxicity, as well as general constitutional approaches described in Chapters 6 – 10, can help. Bodywork, hydrotherapy and deep relaxation are the most useful means of allowing a gradual restoration of well-being.

## Sleep problems

It might be thought that people with muscular pain sleep badly because of the pain, and this is indeed true for many people – that the muscular pain makes it harder to sleep soundly. However, what has emerged from research into fibromyalgia is that the muscular aches and pains are frequently actually the result of the same processes that disturb the sleep pattern. This suggests that imbalances resulting from the poor sleep patterns help to create the muscular symptoms. If this were true it would mean that the poorer the sleep, the more tender points would be found and the greater the fatigue – and research confirms that this is the case. It is now well established that whatever disturbs the sleep and causes a chain reaction of other problems (see below) is usually unrelated to the person's psychological status.

### UNDERSTANDING THE SLEEP PROCESS

In normal sleep, we pass through a series of stages that are characterized by different electrical patterns in the brain – the whole cycle involving all the stages taking around 90 minutes.

We pass through what are known as alpha brain wave patterns (stage 1), which is a light sleep, through progressively deeper stages (stages 2, 3 and 4, or beta, gamma, delta – the deepest period of sleep). The last three stages are also known as non-rapid eye movement (REM) sleep, as the eye movements that occur during dreaming in the first stage are absent in all of the remaining stages.

Sleep laboratories studying people's sleep patterns have found that nearly half of all people with fibromyalgia have disturbed delta stages (that is, intrusive alpha-wave periods occur during them) and tend to wake up feeling as tired as they did when they went to bed, or even more so.

A large percentage of the remainder of fibromyalgia sufferers experience other forms of disturbed sleep (see below).

Prescription antidepressant medications which are sometimes able to reduce many of the symptoms of fibromyalgia include various drugs which, while they increase the amount of sleep sufferers get, have not been shown to alter the disturbed and limited delta stages by more than a small amount.

## THE GROWTH HORMONE CONNECTION

The sleep that is most restful is the delta stage, with 'repairing' hormones (growth hormone) being released by the pituitary gland at this time, as well as immune system repair functions being more active.

Growth hormone, 80 per cent of which is produced during delta-stage sleep, has been shown to have a direct effect on the quality of repair and regeneration of muscles, so that when it is not produced in sufficient amounts because of disturbed sleep, this could account, at least in part, for the muscular symptoms of fibromyalgia.

There is evidence aplenty that growth hormone production can be encouraged by specific dietary strategies (and during deep relaxation or meditation). These methods are discussed in Chapter 6.

## HOW THE MUSCLES ARE AFFECTED

Just how easily disturbed sleep can upset muscular status was demonstrated by Dr. H. Moldofsky in a study in which volunteers had their delta-stage sleep disrupted for three nights in a row (1993).

All the volunteers developed fatigue, widespread aching muscles and specific tenderness on palpation of those sites, indicating a diagnosis of fibromyalgia. Interestingly, when the same sleep disruption pattern was used on volunteer long-distance runners, there was no fatigue and no pain. This suggests that the benefits of aerobic training enhances the way the body can respond to stresses such as sleep deprivation.

As we will see, carefully constructed 'training' can be an effective way of ensuring a recovery from fibromyalgia.

It may be asked why people who suffer 'ordinary' insomnia do not develop fibromyalgia. This has been well researched. Some studies have now shown that 'normal' insomnia does not involve the same degree of disturbance of delta-stage sleep (by alpha waves) that occurs in fibromyalgia. When normal sleep is disturbed by insomnia, there is also often a greater degree of 'arousal' or increased neurological excitability than is evident in fibromyalgia sufferers. In other words, it is a different form of sleep disturbance, and because delta-wave sleep is not upset, growth hormone production remains relatively normal, so muscular dysfunction does not occur as a result of 'ordinary' insomnia.

## 'BRAIN-FOG' AND OTHER SYMPTOMS

Among the obvious, and now proven, effects of disturbed sleep are many of the symptoms often associated with fibromyalgia and chronic fatigue syndrome (ME).

Where delta-stage sleep is artificially disturbed in volunteers, a host of symptoms appear – tiredness, difficulty in concentrating or remembering things, problems in thinking of words, poor ability in doing mental arithmetic or other similar tasks, forgetfulness and so on. Many people affected in this way describe their brains as 'being in a fog'.

When their sleep continues to be disturbed, volunteers have become withdrawn and started to complain of physical symptoms, increased muscular and joint tenderness and stiffness.

All of these physical and mental symptoms disappear when delta-stage sleep is restored for just two nights.

## SEROTONIN
A number of biochemical imbalances can influence sleep patterns – most notably a lack of serotonin. This is a neurotransmitter (neurotransmitters are substances that influence the way nerve messages are passed in the body – either damping them down or boosting them). A deficiency of serotonin can cause depression as well as lower pain thresholds. There are nutritional and other strategies that can help modify neurotransmitter production; these are outlined in Chapter 6.

There is also definite depression of the effectiveness of the immune system during periods of sleep disturbance, and this may account, at least in part, for the continuous viral problems many people with chronic fatigue and fibromyalgia experience.

Bodywork – especially massage, relaxation techniques and hypnotism, acupuncture and hydrotherapy methods – nutritional strategies and specific herbal and homoeopathic medicines can all help ease or resolve sleep problems.

## OTHER SLEEP ANOMALIES
Fibromyalgia sufferers may experience sleep apnoea (a long period during which breathing stops), unpleasant spasms in the arms or legs (nocturnal myoclonus) or tooth grinding (bruxism).

### Sleep apnoea
This occurs in around 25 per cent of fibromyalgia sufferers. The problem is thought to result from the tongue falling back in the

throat, obstructing the airway (much as snoring is caused). Some (very few) people's apnoea seems to be caused by a brain 'error' in the regulation of the breathing muscles (considered to be the cause of sudden infant death syndrome – SIDS – by many experts).

Surgery is sometimes effective in resolving this problem – lifting the oropharynx and/or tongue and so preventing it from falling back during sleep.

A less traumatic treatment is to sew a ping-pong ball on to the back of the nightclothes so that the person will wake up when they turn on to their back, as apnoea doesn't happen when lying on one's side or front!

One of the leading researchers into fibromyalgia, Dr. Harvey Moldofsky, reports that all substances containing caffeine (coffee, tea, chocolate, cola) should be avoided by people with sleep apnoea, as well as alcohol and tricyclic (antidepressant) medication.

### Myoclonus (restless leg syndrome)

This affects about 16 per cent of fibromyalgia sufferers. It should be noted that while antidepressant medication helps restore restful sleep for most other fibromyalgia sufferers, it is not effective for people with nocturnal myoclonus.

Experts such as Daniel Wallace, MD, claim that anticonvulsive medication will return a fibromyalgia sufferer to normal (muscle pain, fatigue and all) within a week if myoclonus is their chief symptom of disturbed sleep (Fibromyalgia Network Newsletters, 1993, 1994).

Nutritional help is also available in the form of folic acid (a B vitamin), vitamin E, and a nutrient known as 5-hydroxy-l-tryptophan (5-HTP) which all assist 'restless leg' symptoms. 5-HTP also helps restore natural sleep patterns, as it is a precursor of serotonin. The avoidance of caffeine is also important if sleep patterns are to be restored. Additional details of nutritional help for FMS/CFS will be found in Chapters 6 and 10 (including more on 5-HTP.)

*Bruxism*

Tooth-grinding affects between 10 and 15 per cent of fibromyalgia sufferers, and is best treated by a dentist or orthodontist who may provide special plates to be worn at night to protect the teeth from damage due to the grinding.

### A CAUTIONARY NOTE ON TREATING DISTURBED SLEEP

A return to a better sleep pattern is clearly a key, some say *the* key, to normalizing or helping people with fibromyalgia, but different treatments are required for different forms of sleep problems!

Whether or not the same benefits gained by taking medication for disturbed sleep can be achieved by more natural means is a question that is considered in later sections of this book.

### Tempero-mandibular joint (TMJ) problems

See Bruxism, above, and Chapter 3.

### Thyroid

Some researchers believe that all the symptoms of FMS can be accounted for by thyroid gland dysfunction. Whether this is completely true or not, it is now certain that a great many people with FMS have, as an underlying feature of their problem, an imbalance in their thyroid hormone function, even though they may have apparently normal levels of thyroid hormone in their bloodstream.

This is an important distinction. The person may be producing 'normal' levels of thyroid hormone . . . but its function may not be adequate; the hormone may be only partially active. In such a case, having a thyroid function test may not pick up the problem. Test results may show normal levels of circulating thyroid hormones, and so your physician might dismiss the idea that FMS is linked to thyroid deficiency. The sad truth is that there are times when the cells to which the hormones have to attach in order to become active, resist the attachment. This is known as 'partial cellular resistance', which may result from a number of causes (something similar happens in diabetes in some cases, where insulin is present but cannot become active because of 'cellular resistance').

Why should this happen? Why should cells of the body which need it, resist the attachment of thyroid hormones?

Several reasons are known:

- Genetic predisposition. Mutations of chromosomes have been shown to be one reason, and can sometimes result from radiation exposure.
- Deficiency, especially of B-complex vitamins, can reduce the efficiency of thyroid function.
- Toxicity involving widely distributed toxic substances such as polychlorinated biphenyls (PCBs), dioxin and DDT can interfere with normal thyroid hormone function. Another mechanism is thought to involve these toxins, causing increased liver excretion of thyroid hormone.
- Medications such as beta blockers can also interfere with thyroid hormone function.
- Allergy or autoimmune factors may play a part in why thyroid hormone cannot perform its normal tasks.
- Active exercise to aerobic levels seems to encourage thyroid hormone function; conversely, lack of activity may retard such function.

Research has confirmed many of the connections between thyroid deficiency/thyroid hormone dysfunction and the symptoms of fibromyalgia, chronic muscle pain and chronic fatigue:

- The symptoms of fibromyalgia closely resemble those of underactive thyroid function (producing insufficient levels of thyroid hormone production) including depression, mental fatigue, anxiety, poor memory, sleep disturbance, headaches, gastrointestinal dysfunction, menstrual irregularities, fatigue, hypoglycaemia, sensitivity to cold, increased susceptibility to infection, musculoskeletal symptoms and skin problems (S. Wilke, 1981, L. Sonkin, 1985).

- Many fibromyalgia patients have as an associated condition hypothyroidism (underactive thyroid) (G. Ferraccioli, 1990).
- John Lowe DC, and colleagues, suggest that when thyroid function is apparently normal (euthyroid) in patients with FMS, the FMS may be the result of a failure of normal thyroid hormone to function correctly due to 'cellular resistance' to the hormone (J. Lowe, 1997).
- Lowe (1997) conducted a study in which metabolic rehabilitation (the term he uses for his thyroid hormone treatment method) was shown to be long lasting, for years after thyroid hormone supplementation ceased. When fibromyalgia patients who had received the thyroid treatment were compared with those who had not, after up to five years there was a marked difference in all symptoms as well as in the use of medications such as antidepressants and pain and anti-inflammatory drugs. These results show that the benefits of thyroid supplementation (when it is indicated) are not due to placebo effects and are long lasting.
- Other trials support the use of thyroid treatment, with fibromyalgia patients improving dramatically following suitable thyroid replacement and other supportive strategies (see below) without side-effects, it is claimed (J. Lowe et al., 1997).
- Norwegian research has shown that there is a frequent incidence of thyroid dysfunction in people (especially women) who have fibromyalgia. This is not picked up when normal thyroid function tests are done, but shows up when antibodies to thyroid hormone are tested for. What this means is that these individuals may be producing adequate thyroid hormone but, for reasons

which are not entirely clear, their immune systems are deactivating this, giving an appearance of normal thyroid function but with the symptoms (including widespread muscle pain) of underactive thyroid (T. Aarflot, 1996).

■ Chronic muscle pain resulting from the activity of myofascial trigger points (see Chapter 4) is more severe when thyroid hormone and B vitamins are deficient, according to the main researchers into this, Drs Travell and Simons (1998).There is an overlap in the pain which comes from FMS and that which comes from myofascial pain syndrome (MFS), quite different conditions which may coexist in the same person. Both conditions would be aggravated by thyroid imbalance.

## Thyroid imbalance questionnaire and test ❓

The following tests and questions should help you to determine whether there is a possibility of an underactive thyroid, or of thyroid hormone dysfunction. If the results of the questionnaire and the test support each other (that is, they both suggest underactive thyroid function), you should seek out a suitably qualified physician who can help you to rebalance and rehabilitate this vital function. Further information will be found in Chapter 6.

| 1 | Does your weight increase easily? |
|---|---|
| 2 | Do you get tired very easily and/or feel fatigued most of the time? |
| 3 | Do you have dry skin? |
| 4 | Are you sensitive to the cold? |
| 5 | Are you losing your hair and/or is your hair coarse? |
| 6 | Do you have a poor appetite? |
| 7 | Are the outer thirds of your eyebrows thinning? |
| 8 | Is your resting pulse below 65 beats per minute? |

If you answered YES to at least three of these questions, including at least two of the first four questions, then an underactive thyroid is a real possibility. It is important to remember, however, that there are many other reasons for all or any of these symptoms, other than thyroid dysfunction.

To add to the evidence you are collecting, the 'underarm temperature test' is suggested.

### The Barnes' underarm temperature test

This test looks at what your core temperature is, representing as it does your current metabolic activity (which is to a large extent dependent on thyroid function). Look back at the list of symptoms that Dr. Jessop found in her more than 1,300 fibromyalgia/chronic fatigue patients (page 16), which showed that 65 per cent had below-normal temperature levels!

- Obtain a mercury body thermometer (not an electronic one) and, after shaking it down below 96°F/35°C, place it next your bed so that it can be used first thing on waking.
- On waking, before you get out of bed and before eating or drinking anything, place the thermometer under your arm and leave it in place for *10 minutes*. Lie and rest during this period, moving as little as possible.
- Read the temperature and record this, together with the date. Do the same thing for three mornings in a row.
- If you are a woman and are still menstruating, perform the test on days 2, 3 and 4 of your period.
- Add the totals for the three days together, and divide by three for an average. If this average is below 97.2°F (36.2°C), there is a very strong possibility of an underactive thyroid function being involved.

Strategies to assist thyroid function will be found in Chapters 3 and 6.

## Viral connections

There has long been a suggested connection between viral infections and chronic fatigue syndrome (ME) – indeed, the latter was once called Epstein-Barr disease and is often still termed post-viral fatigue syndrome. Chances are that whatever it is that causes the immune system to become depressed enough to allow a constant viral activity also causes many of the symptoms of fibromyalgia and chronic fatigue syndrome (ME) – probably involving a combination of allergies, toxicity, deficiency, stress and so on. Latent viruses can become active, and in turn start including 'flu-like' symptoms of aches and pains, due to the release of chemicals called cytokines. The virus in such a situation is simply taking the opportunity of disturbed immune function to proliferate, and is not the cause of the problem.

Dr. Anne Macintyre offers research evidence for this, and states, 'The onset of M.E. usually seems to be triggered by a virus, though the infection may pass unnoticed (J. Gow, 1991) . . . Many people say they were fit and well before a viral infection which started their M.E. [FMS] but it is possible that in many such patients there have been other factors such as emotional stress, pesticide exposure, surgical or accidental trauma [see Whiplash, below], some months before the triggering infection' (A. Macintyre, 1993).

Dr. Goldenberg is clear that, 'it is unlikely that a single infection is the cause of most cases of fibromyalgia. Studies of the complicated integration of mind, body and patient's psychological milieu are more likely to provide meaningful answers to all potential factors, including infections, that may be associated with fibromyalgia' (D. Goldenberg, 1994).

Dr. Macintyre (A. Macintyre, 1993), herself afflicted with ME, writes, 'The incidence of new cases peaks in late summer and autumn, coincident with the peak time of year for enteroviral infections. It is likely that enteroviral infection accounts for the majority of M.E. illness in this country [UK], even if other factors (stress, trauma) are present. There may also be a genetic predisposition, evidenced by the higher than expected number of parents with M.E. whose children also develop it some years after the parents' (E.Dowsett, 1990).

Some of the major (possible) influences of viral infections on FMS are summarized below.

- HHV6, one of the herpes viruses, is more commonly found in FMS/CFS patients than other people (D. Buchwald *et al.*, 1992).
- British research which examined stool samples and blood evidence implicates enteroviruses (P. Behan, 1993, J. Gow, 1991).
- Buskila and Simms have both reported on the presence of FMS symptoms in patients infected by HIV (D. Buskila, 1990, R. Simms, 1992).
- Chronic coxsackie B virus infection has been shown to mimic FMS symptoms (P. Nash, 1989).
- Parvovirus has likewise been associated with FMS (L. Leventhal, 1991).

To date, there is certainly no single virus connected with chronic fatigue syndrome (ME) and fibromyalgia, although work continues in search of an elusive culprit on whom to blame these widespread conditions.

Focusing on enhancing immune function through sound nutrition, reduced stress levels and environmental stressors (pollutants and so on) would seem to be a far more positive approach, as it is a weakness of the defence system that allows viral activity to develop in the first place.

### Whiplash

During whiplash injury the head is thrown forwards, backwards or sideways (usually a combination of all of these movements) extremely violently, often causing major damage to nerves and muscles at the base of the skull. One hundred patients with whiplash injury, and also approximately 60 patients with leg trauma (such as fracture), were studied for the presence of severe pain (such as fibromyalgia syndrome) a year after their accidents (D. Buskila *et al.*, 1997).

The findings were that people with neck injuries of this sort were 13 times more likely to develop fibromyalgia than those with severe leg injuries. Fully 21 per cent of those who had experienced whiplash had fibromyalgia within 3.2 months of the accident, while fewer than 2 per cent of those who had leg injuries had this diagnosis. The neck injury patients had lower pain thresholds, more 'tender' points and worse quality of life.

Why should a whiplash-type injury provoke FMS more effectively than other forms of trauma? One answer may lie in a particular muscle at the base of the neck – this will be discussed in Chapter 4.

# 3

# Fibromyalgia – What It Is and What It Is Not

While widespread pain is its most obvious symptom, fibromyalgia is not just a condition involving muscular pain – it always has associated with it a number of other health problems, some of which give us clues as to how the problem started and is maintained. These other problems help to emphasize the fact that fibromyalgia does not have a single cause, but is almost always the end result of several, sometimes numerous interacting causes, with evidence accumulating that there may indeed be a genetic predisposition towards its development. Whether or not you inherited a genetic tendency towards fibromyalgia, and while it can exist alone, it more usually occurs alongside one or more of the conditions examined in Chapter 2.

As muscular pain can be a symptom of many other conditions and diseases, it is absolutely vital that these other conditions are ruled out (or confirmed) before a diagnosis of fibromyalgia is considered. For this reason, in this chapter we shall see what fibromyalgia is *not* by looking at some of the conditions with which it can be confused. These are:

- ankylosing spondylitis
- arthritic conditions
- bacterial endocarditis and acute pericarditis
- calcium metabolism disorders
- carpal tunnel syndrome
- hyperthyroidism and hypothyroidism (see Chapters 2 and 6)
- local muscular problems (see Chapter 4)
- lupus erythematosus
- neurological diseases
- overuse and tempero-mandibular joint syndromes Parkinson's disease
- polymyalgia rheumatica
- polymyositis
- psychogenic rheumatic disorders reflex
- sympathetic dystrophy
- Sjögren'ssyndrome
- viral infections.

## Some conditions which can be confused with fibromyalgia

### ANKYLOSING SPONDYLITIS

The early symptoms of this slow, progressive, degenerative autoimmune condition are recurrent lower back pain, pain along the sciatic nerve and stiffness in the morning. It affects mainly young men and its progression involves the symptoms spreading to the neck and middle and/or upper back, the person affected being locked in a forward bending position ('bamboo spine'). Fatigue is a common feature, as are weight loss, extreme muscle stiffness and anaemia.

This is an autoimmune response in which the body attacks part of itself. This may be because the immune system wrongly identifies itself as a particular invading organism commonly found in the intestines of people with this condition (*Klebsiella*) and attacks itself in the confusion. This is thought to be because the type of protein construction ('protein type') of *Klebsiella* is similar to that of most people who develop ankylosing spondylitis. A similar case of mistaken identity is thought by some researchers to be involved in the start of rheumatoid arthritis (this time involving the bacteria *Proteus*). Rheumatology testing can establish a diagnosis of ankylosing spondylitis fairly rapidly and distinguish it from fibromyalgia in the process.

## ARTHRITIC CONDITIONS

Conditions such as osteoarthritis and rheumatoid arthritis commonly exist alongside fibromyalgia but cannot themselves be confused with it. Blood tests and other clinical investigation techniques can usually show what type of rheumatic condition is present and whether or not this is responsible for whatever pain is being reported. As mentioned above, someone with one of these conditions can also have fibromyalgia, and this should be appropriately examined and investigated if the pain being reported does not fit with the rheumatic disorder alone.

### Lyme disease

This is often mistakenly diagnosed when fibromyalgia is in fact the problem. If a patient with Lyme disease has not responded to conventional antibiotic therapy for this tick-borne infectious disease, or if the person has responded but continues to have pain, then fibromyalgia should be seriously considered as being the explanation for this.

## BACTERIAL ENDOCARDITIS AND ACUTE PERICARDITIS

Acute endocarditis is characterized by fever, excessive perspiration, periodic rigors (extreme spasm-like episodes) and usually follows on from an infection such as pneumonia or a septic wound. In acute pericarditis the patient is anxious, the cheeks are pale, the face is puffy and there is fever, a rapid pulse and rapid breathing with, commonly, pain in the chest (on the left side mostly) and sometimes the abdomen. There is often a cough, too. Immediate emergency medical attention is required.

It is hard to see how these conditions could be confused with fibromyalgia, but they are listed as needing to be ruled out by many experts.

## CALCIUM METABOLISM DISORDERS

Calcium is one of the main bulk minerals needed by the body – almost all (99 per cent) of it being used in the bones and teeth. The small amount not needed for these purposes is used by the body in many essential biochemical processes.

If a parathyroid hormone imbalance exists (with the gland producing too much as a rule), a chain reaction of events can occur leading to decalcification of bone and this calcium being deposited in the soft tissues instead. This chain reaction can be further complicated by menopausal and other hormonal disturbances – especially when oestrogen levels drop. Among the negative influences such changes can produce are bone pains, psychiatric symptoms (most notably anxiety, nervous tics, insomnia, hyperactivity and panic attacks) as well as constipation – all of which, as we have seen, may occur in chronic fatigue syndrome (ME) and fibromyalgia.

Parathyroid overactivity is treatable surgically as well as through nutritional therapy.

Calcium deficiency can produce the same symptoms as parathyroid overactivity. Supplementation with calcium (1,000 to 1,500 mg daily and/or increased dietary intake) can usually correct this.

If someone has poor muscle tone, constipation, abdominal pains, loss of appetite, vomiting and muscular pains, investigation into the functioning of their parathyroid and calcium-absorbing systems is required. It would also be useful for levels of digestive acids to be tested as these can be low, resulting in poor calcium absorption.

Magnesium supplementation is also often useful in helping to normalize calcium metabolism disturbance, as it counters excessive levels of parathyroid hormone in the body and encourages calcium deposition in bones, as well as the removal of excess calcium from muscle.

It is not uncommon for people with fibromyalgia-like symptoms to have some degree of calcium (or magnesium) imbalance and, in many instances, this could be part of the underlying complex of causes of the problem. General supplementation details are to be found in Chapter 6. Dr. John Lowe recommends 'a minimum' of 1 gram of magnesium and 2 grams of calcium, to be supplemented daily for all fibromyalgia patients (Lowe 1999).

## CARPAL TUNNEL SYNDROME

This local, painful hand and wrist condition is caused by some degree of compression of the median nerve as it passes through the tunnel of bones at the wrist – causing tingling, pain, stiffness, numbness and, sometimes, weakness (most commonly in the thumb, index and middle fingers). The symptoms may even wake the sufferer at night. This may result from repetitive use – as in typing.

Various specific nerve conduction tests can identify interference with nerve transmission; this sort of test may be helpful in proving whether or not a trapped nerve is part of the problem, as many people with fibromyalgia have symptoms that mimic those of carpal tunnel syndrome. Another form of pressure on these nerves can be caused by fluid retention (such as occurs during pregnancy).

Steroids or surgery are the most common suggestions doctors have for treating the problem. However, manipulation, acupuncture and supplementation with vitamin $B_6$ are reported to help normalize the situation.

Carpal tunnel syndrome is a local arm and hand problem and not a generalized condition like fibromyalgia. This said, it can of course be present in someone with fibromyalgia and be responsible for some of the pain being reported. Whether this is the case or not should be assessed by an expert. Manual treatment which releases the short tight muscles of the arm, and which balances and releases muscles and joints in the upper spine, neck and shoulders, can often correct the biomechanical problems associated with carpal tunnel syndrome. Trigger point deactivation may also be necessary (see Chapter 4). In some cases surgical decompression is necessary to achieve relief.

## HYPERTHYROIDISM AND HYPOTHYROIDISM

Fatigue is commonly a feature of an overactive thyroid (hyperthyroidism), as are anxiety, gastrointestinal disturbances and chest pain. As we have seen, these symptoms are also common in fibromyalgia. However, other symptoms of an overactive thyroid, such as tremors, wide (bulging) staring eyes, agitation, weight loss, excessive sweating, low tolerance of heat and increased appetite are less likely to occur in fibromyalgia.

There is now a great deal of evidence that an underactive thyroid (hypothyroidism) may be involved in some instances of fibromyalgia. While many doctors insist that blood tests can give a clear indication as to whether or not hyper – or hypothyroidism are the causes of the problems, this is disputed by researchers such as Dr. John Lowe (1998, 1999). He reports that in many hundreds of fibromyalgia patients who had symptoms which closely resembled underactive thyroid (see questionnaire in Chapter 2), he found that an average of around 40 per cent appeared (based on blood tests) to have normal thyroid function, but nevertheless responded well to thyroid treatment.

### Why should there be underactive thyroid hormone function?
The reasons why someone who has a blood test which shows adequate levels of the active thyroid hormone (T3), but who seems to need way above normal levels in order to function normally, include the following possibilities:

- autoimmune thyroiditis (which may result from radiation exposure)
- surgical removal of part of the thyroid
- pituitary gland dysfunction
- interference with normal thyroid hormone function by toxins such as dioxin or PCBs
- interference with normal thyroid hormone function due to particular medication such as beta blockers
- interference with normal thyroid hormone function due to particular nutritional deficiencies such as B-complex
- interference with normal thyroid hormone function due to an allergic response
- genetic defects (mutation of chromosome 3) which produces 'cellular resistance' to thyroid hormone, preventing it from working normally.

All or any of these causes, and possibly others, might create a situation in which thyroid hormone was not being produced adequately or converted adequately, or was not working adequately. All of these situations would lead to symptoms which in many particulars look *exactly like fibromyalgia*.

### What can be done about this type of thyroid dysfunction?

1 Find a sympathetic and understanding physician who is prepared to work carefully towards normalization of thyroid function (see the Useful Publications and Addresses section at the end of this book for support group details).
2 Avoid or try to modify any of the possible 'causes' listed above (toxicity, deficiency, allergy, etc.). See Chapter 6 for suggestions as to how to start these processes.

3   Get more exercise. There is evidence that
    physiological activity such as aerobic exercise
    helps thyroid function. Inactivity should be
    avoided if at all possible.

Dietary suggestions to assist thyroid function will be found in Chapter 6.

## LUPUS ERYTHEMATOSUS

Systemic lupus erythematosus is a chronic inflammatory disease and an autoimmune condition in which the immune system attacks parts of the body it is supposed to be defending. Its symptoms include fatigue as a key early sign, as well as arthritis-like joint pains, and swellings, fever and skin lesions which are often over the face ('butterfly rash'). Fibrositis-like muscle pains are also usually present. Sensitivity to sunlight is often noted, as is hair loss. Cold extremities are another feature, which is also common to many people with fibromyalgia. It affects young women almost exclusively and occurs more frequently in people of African descent than in Caucasian peoples.

Anti-inflammatory painkilling medication is usually effective in combating the symptoms – unlike in fibromyalgia – especially in the early stages or in mild forms. When the disease is more active, steroid medication, antibiotics and immunosuppressive drugs are used with varying degrees of success.

A check-up carried out by a rheumatologist is needed to establish a diagnosis of lupus (the presence of antinuclear antibodies, for example), which is not easy to diagnose for certain in the early stages. Also, spontaneous remission is not uncommon.

## NEUROLOGICAL DISEASES

### Multiple sclerosis (MS)

This disease affects the central nervous system, leading, initially, to pins and needles sensations in the hands and/or feet, numbness, loss of balance, clumsiness, sensitivity to both heat and cold, blurred or double vision and difficulty in walking. In its advanced stages, movements become jerky, muscles become increasingly weak, speech slurs and urinary urgency or incontinence can appear. Intense fatigue is also a common feature.

A neurological examination is needed to diagnose someone as having MS.

### Neuropathy

This is a general term for disturbances and pathologies of the peripheral nervous system, and symptoms of tingling, weakness and pain are the usual result. Again, a neurological examination is needed to make a definite diagnosis.

## OVERUSE AND TEMPERO-MANDIBULAR JOINT (TMJ) SYNDROMES

Occupational and habitual overuse of particular areas of the body can result in chronically altered biomechanics and pain. The difference between such conditions and fibromyalgia will be that in these other conditions the nature of the problem will be a localized rather than widespread presence of tender points and pain. It is not uncommon for someone with fibromyalgia to have a pattern of overuse as well, and expert analysis of the pain and the history should be able to identify this.

Appropriate medicine and manipulative bodywork, along with reeducation as to how to use the body less stressfully, is usually helpful in normalizing overuse syndrome problems.

Tempera-mandibular joint syndrome problems can be the result of localized injuries (dental work or traumatic impacts, such as a blow), or the end result of postural imbalances which end up as localized muscular and joint stress focused on and felt in the jaw region, causing pain on chewing or opening the mouth. TMJ syndrome can also result from unbalanced occlusion – a failure of the teeth to meet correctly when chewing or closing the mouth.

The pain of this syndrome, which commonly involves the active presence of myofascial trigger points (see Chapter 4), is usually confined to the head, neck and face rather than the more generalized pattern that goes with fibromyalgia. Neuro-Muscular Therapists (NMT), massage therapists and many other bodywork professionals are trained to find and treat the imbalances which lead to trigger point activity.

As with overuse syndrome, TMJ syndrome problems can coexist, as a part of the fibromyalgia pain picture, along with the other symptoms of FMS. The official estimate is that facial pain affects about 25 per cent of fibromyalgia sufferers. Some of it may involve tempero-mandibular joint syndrome, some not. The cause of pain in the head, face and jaw should be investigated by an expert in manual medicine, a craniosacral therapist and/or a dental expert familiar with these methods. Many osteopaths and chiropractors (and an increasing number of dentists) have focused attention on TMJ problems. These practitioners use variations on cranial manipulation methods (in osteopathy this may be called 'cranial osteopathy' or 'craniosacral therapy', while in chiropractic it may be known as 'sacra-occipital technique'[SOT]).

PARKINSON'S DISEASE

In about 75 per cent of people who develop the condition, the early signs of Parkinson's are of a tremor, usually in one hand (as though rolling something between the fingers), which is worse at rest and less so on movement. Walking becomes a shuffle and other parts of the body can also tremble. Stiffness and muscular rigidity, slowness of movement, resting tremors and postural imbalance are the key signs. Depression and dementia may also occur – men being more susceptible to this than women. The differences between fibromyalgia and Parkinson's are very clear and it should not be difficult to identify which condition the person has.

## POLYMYALGIA RHEUMATICA

This usually affects the elderly (those over 60) and is characterized by marked pain and stiffness in the neck, shoulder and hip regions, starting and progressing rapidly. Morning stiffness is also a feature. Previously called 'muscular rheumatism', it is doubtless sometimes misdiagnosed as fibromyalgia and vice versa. It affects women four times more frequently than men. Blood tests show a raised sedimentation rate (that is, raised levels of 'debris' are found, as a result of inflammations or chronic infection) and sometimes anaemia.

The condition is linked to temporal arteritis (a condition characterized by inflammation of the temporal and other arteries in the head) in many cases, either following on from polymyalgia rheumatica or preceding it.

The symptoms respond dramatically quickly to cortisone medication – unlike fibromyalgia – and blood tests would give a strong indication to the expert examining the sufferer as to which condition he or she had.

## POLYMYOSITIS

This term simply means widespread inflammation and weakness in the voluntary muscles (those under conscious control). If a skin rash (usually a reddish-purple discoloration affecting the eyelids, face and fingers) accompanies the condition, it is called dermatomyositis.

This condition may start at any age, and is more common in women. The early signs are weakness and pain, but it may progress to the muscles that control breathing, with disastrous results. The affected muscles eventually weaken, waste and contract. A link with cancer is found in around 20 per cent of cases.

When the condition occurs in children, the symptoms are cold fingers and ulceration of the skin, with calcified deposits developing under the skin.

Like polymyalgia rheumatica, this condition often responds to steroid medication – unlike fibromyalgia.

## PSYCHOGENIC RHEUMATIC DISORDERS

There was a time – largely in the 1950s but still continuing in some quarters – when muscular pain was not regarded as having a physical or organic cause, and that it was therefore 'psychogenic', that is, all in the mind. The reason this view was held may have been due to a failure on the part of most rheumatologists at that time (and some today) to adequately handle such symptoms, leading to their happily discarding the problem with this phrase, 'it's all in the mind'.

It is true that a great many somatic (of the body) symptoms can indeed result from emotional and psychological causes. For example, depression can involve both pain and fatigue as prominent symptoms, and it is therefore necessary to exclude the possibility that depression might be part of the cause of the pain-fatigue symptoms.

My own experience is that it is unusual for anyone who is severely depressed to muster the energy, or to be bothered even, to ask for help. This suggests that a patient who takes the trouble to look for assistance is probably not clinically depressed, but rather could simply be depressed because of the misery of their symptoms and the lack of interest displayed by their medical advisers (this being reactive depression).

The imagined stigma of having symptoms blamed partially or totally on psychological causes should not prevent us from accepting that, in almost all conditions – from the common cold to cancer – there are bound to be elements of emotional involvement, and that good stress-coping strategies and a balanced emotional outlook can help all conditions, including chronic fatigue syndrome (ME) and fibromyalgia. At its simplest, the mind affects the immune, defence and repair (homeostatic) mechanisms of the body, and these need all the help they can get in fibromyalgia and chronic fatigue syndrome (ME).

There are undoubtedly times when for reasons of great emotional distress a phenomenon known as somatization occurs. When this happens, psychologically-induced symptoms of pain may develop. This sort of event is an established medical occurrence, and when this occurs psychotherapy is called for.

Help from counsellors or psychotherapists can be an invaluable part of a team approach to achieving recovery to full health for those in great pain from any cause. However, it is seldom *just* the mind that needs to be helped in cases of fibromyalgia and chronic fatigue syndrome (ME).

## REFLEX SYMPATHETIC DYSTROPHY

Overactivity of parts of the sympathetic nervous system leads to an intense burning type of pain. The causes range from damage to nerves themselves through trauma to heart attacks and strokes. Sometimes quite minor injuries, such as sprains, lacerations or bone injuries, can trigger this most unpleasant form of incessant pain and extreme local sensitivity. Other symptoms include a form of tissue swelling (oedema) on which finger pressure fails to leave a depression. The skin over the affected area is likely to be very cold, bluish in colour and sweaty, with a tendency to 'goose flesh'.

Diagnosis of this condition is made by means of the medical history of the person, their symptoms and the results of tests, such as thermography (photographs of the areas taken using heat-sensitive film) to see if a characteristic pattern forms. Unlike fibromyalgia, the symptoms of this condition are localized, affecting just one limb, for example.

Some of the symptoms of reflex sympathetic dystrophy can be similar to the effects of active myofascial trigger points and, if this is the case, they need to be carefully evaluated and treated (see Chapter 4).

As with other pain problems, it is possible that someone with fibromyalgia could also have this condition; the possibility of this should be checked out by an expert.

## SJÖGREN'S SYNDROME

This rheumatic condition (its symptoms are similar to those of rheumatoid arthritis) affects mainly middle-aged females and is characterized by dryness of the mucous membranes – mostly affecting the eyes, nose and mouth. The glands that produce saliva are enlarged and the sufferer's appetite is poor.

To differentiate this syndrome from fibromyalgia, blood tests would be done to check for evidence of auto-antibodies and, most obviously, checking whether or not the joints or the muscles are affected, as this condition involves painful joints rather than muscles in the main.

## VIRAL INFECTIONS

See also Chapter 2.

A host of viral infections have been suggested as being related to chronic fatigue syndrome (ME) and fibromyalgia, but there has been no consistent evidence or proof of a causal link. The fact that various viruses are sometimes present (enteroviruses, various herpes viruses, retroviruses and so on) in sufficient numbers to cause symptoms, at the same time as someone has fibromyalgia, does not prove a direct causal link. It is more likely that both conditions (fibromyalgia and viral infections) are the result of an imbalance in the defence mechanisms of the body. Certainly, viral activity can result in cytokine (a biochemical byproduct of viral activity) production, which causes many of the flu-like and pain symptoms so obvious in fibromyalgia. The focus of attention by doctors on the virus tends to distract attention away from efforts to improve immune function so that it can take care of invading organisms as it was designed to do.

Viral infections can therefore exist before, and contribute to, fibromyalgia and chronic fatigue syndrome (ME) problems, and ongoing viral activity can certainly be a part of the cause of the symptom picture, deserving some attention. However, the focus should be on immune system enhancement, as outlined in other chapters.

### Screening tests for fibromyalgia and chronic fatigue syndrome (ME)

It is certainly not uncommon for someone with either of the major symptom patterns we are considering – chronic fatigue and/or chronic muscular pain – to undergo a battery of tests that prove negative or borderline at best. The truth is that, at present, there are no absolute diagnostic laboratory tests for these conditions, only ones that rule out other conditions or suggest a possible diagnosis.

A far more satisfactory method of finding out what is going on is to use old-fashioned, low-tech interview, case history, examination and palpation (feeling the body by hand) methods, supported by tests that rule out other possible causes and help the practitioner to come to a diagnosis of what it is by a process of elimination.

Among the most common are:

- blood tests
- nutritional evaluation tests
- X-rays
- brain scans
- electrical conduction tests
- muscle enzyme assessments
- analysis of stool samples
- thermography
- palpation.

Let us look at each of these in more detail.

## BLOOD TESTS

These can determine:

- blood status – whether or not there are normal levels and ratios of the various blood cells
- the presence of infectious agents or their markers (substances produced if the immune system has dealt, or is dealing, with them)
- nutritional status – which nutrients are in the bloodstream, and at what levels, although the test can give only a rough idea as to the general nutritional status (there are more accurate ways of checking the nutritional status of the body as a whole, rather than just looking at the blood)
- evidence that there is low (or high) levels of thyroid hormone, although this will not determine whether the hormonal function is normal. See discussions of the thyroid above and in Chapter 2
- iron levels (anaemia is diagnosed if the levels are too low)
- indication of allergic response
- evidence of specific infections (current or past), as there will be antibodies for such infections as Lyme disease, Epstein-Barr virus or one of the herpes viruses, and the level of concentration of the antibody can indicate whether or not the immune system is overreacting to a previous or current infection, something that is not uncommon in chronic fatigue syndrome (ME) and fibromyalgia sufferers
- presence of rheumatoid factor, which shows that the person tested may have rheumatoid arthritis (false positive tests are not uncommon in normal individuals, but this test is almost always positive when there is rheumatoid arthritis)

- high erythrocyte sedimentation rate, which indicates that there is probably an active infection or inflammation in the body – a high reading is likely if there is polymyalgia rheumatica, rheumatoid arthritis, lupus or some such chronic systemic condition, but levels in fibromyalgia patients are usually normal
- the presence of antinuclear antibodies, which is discovered by assessing how the nuclei of healthy cells respond to antibodies – when the count is high it is considered that an autoimmune condition is present (Sjögren's syndrome, lupus erythematosus, ankylosing spondylitis, rheumatoid arthritis and so on). Between 15 and 20 per cent of people with fibromyalgia have a high antinuclear antibody count, although it is also found to be higher than normal in many apparently healthy elderly people.

## NUTRITIONAL EVALUATION TESTS

These can be carried out using blood tests, sweat tests, hair analysis, computer programmes, eating diaries – all of which can give clues as to what levels of specific nutrient imbalances might exist. There are major areas of disagreement among experts as to the validity and relevance of the many ways there are to try to evaluate a person's nutritional status.

## X-RAYS

These are completely useless in helping to identify fibromyalgia. However, they can show arthritic and other degenerative changes in joints, which can help to explain some of the pain being felt. Most people over 40, though, have some arthritic changes in their spines, especially in their necks, and most are pain-free despite these changes.

## BRAIN SCANS

Various forms of scan are capable of showing specific patterns of lowered blood circulation through parts of the brain, which seem to be a hallmark of chronic fatigue syndrome (ME) and fibromyalgia. MRI and CAT scans can also rule out the presence of multiple sclerosis, which involves damage to the sheaths in which nerves are enclosed. These tests are very expensive.

## ELECTRICAL CONDUCTION TESTS

These can be used to find out how well nerves are transmitting their impulses. They are most useful in differentiating pain, numbness and tingling in the extremities, such as occur when there is either carpal tunnel syndrome (symptoms in the wrist and hand) or thoracic inlet syndrome (involving the whole arm). Such sensations can be a part of the pain experienced by someone with fibromyalgia, but these tests cannot delineate the generalized symptom picture. Neurologists use these tests to establish particular patterns of dysfunction.

## MUSCLE ENZYME ASSESSMENTS

These differentiate between fibromyalgia and muscular dystrophy. Samples of muscle tissue may need to be removed for assessment of the presence of specific enzymes. The results will be normal for anyone with fibromyalgia.

## ANALYSIS OF STOOL SAMPLES

This can be useful when trying to identify whether or not there is any yeast, bacterial or parasitic activity present. Sophisticated stool analysis can now be conducted to offer a wide range of evidence which nutritionists, herbalists, naturopaths, chiropractors and some physicians find useful in deciding on treatment strategies, and for monitoring progress.

Other ways of identifying yeast activity include a sugar-loading test, which involves assessing levels of blood alcohol before and after a high sugar intake. Yeasts (and some bacteria) turn sugar into alcohol, and the dramatic rise in blood alcohol levels this test can produce, along with a host of symptoms including 'brain fog' in many cases, is impressive enough to cause many patients to abandon their sugar-bingeing.

## THERMOGRAPHY

The body's surface is filmed or photographed using heat-sensitive apparatus and film that shows up hot and cold areas. The results can be used to identify the presence of trigger points and areas of active inflammation – there should be no inflammation in fibromyalgia, whereas trigger points may show up as 'hot-spots' (although trigger points are sometimes in fibrotic tissues with poor circulation, and so may appear 'cold').

## PALPATION

Touching and feeling the appropriate tender point sites is the acceptable method for identifying fibromyalgia. If the points (11 out of 18) are reported to be sensitive – using a standard degree of finger or thumb pressure (not more than 4 kg/8 ¾ lb), then this indicates that the person has fibromyalgia. A small rubber-tipped pressure gauge, known as an algometer, is sometimes used when applying pressure so that the exact amount of pressure needed to produce the pain can be measured.

## What abnormalities point to a diagnosis of fibromyalgia?

### DISTURBED SLEEP PATTERNS

Experts in sleep disorders can look at such patterns and evaluate just how much alpha brain wave disturbance of the delta sleep periods there is. This is one of the most accepted (medically) characteristics of fibromyalgia and goes some way to explaining the sequence of events that ends with pain in the muscles (see Chapter 2, page 15).

A sleep laboratory is required for such tests, which makes this an expensive or difficult assessment to obtain, unless the individual is lucky enough to be part of a research project!

## LOW GROWTH HORMONE LEVELS

These will be evident (confirmed by specialized blood tests) if there is an underactive pituitary gland or if the disturbed sleep affects delta sleep patterns (when growth hormone is secreted). There are strategies for helping to stimulate growth hormone production, described in Chapter 6.

## IMBALANCES IN NEUROTRANSMITTER LEVELS

These will be apparent in many people with fibromyalgia, especially in relation to low serotonin, dopamine and/or epinephrine levels and/or excessive levels of substance P. These influence our sleep patterns and how strongly we register pain. Blood tests can provide evidence of such imbalances.

## AMINO ACID IMBALANCES

These can be expected in many people with fibromyalgia. Amino acids are the building units of different proteins, the raw materials for the production of vital chemicals in the body, such as serotonin (and, therefore, the important substances that derive from it – dopamine and epinephrine). All these are manufactured in the body from the amino acid tryptophan, which is commonly found to be in short supply in people with fibromyalgia. There are a number of ways of assessing amino acid status, including blood and urine tests.

Various nutritional strategies involving this and other amino acids are given in Chapter 6.

## IMMUNE SYSTEM IMBALANCES AND DEFICIENCIES

These are found in some people with fibromyalgia, and measurement of what is called 'natural killer cell activity' can be carried out following blood tests.

## COLLAGEN SYNTHESIS DYSFUNCTION

This can be a part of the problem for some people with both fibromyalgia and a tendency towards hypermobility of the joints. Collagen is the basic substance used by the body to build connective tissue, which is the stabilizing 'cement' of the body. Special blood tests can identify imbalances in the process by which collagen is manufactured in the body, particularly where there is a low concentration of a substance called pro-collagen type III amino-terminal peptide – or PIIINP for short.

### The way forward

Research continues into these and other specific areas of interest to fibromyalgia and chronic fatigue syndrome (ME) sufferers, and, as it does, we are learning more and more about the biochemical imbalances which occur in the muscles and other tissues of people who are affected.

It is worth restating that, in trying to get well again, our focus should be on several fronts at the same time, removing causes wherever these can be discovered. This might involve lowering stress levels, enhancing nutritional balance, metabolic rehabilitation (for example, by normalizing thyroid function), detoxifying, avoiding allergens and so on. At the same time, general, constitutional, non-specific immune-enhancing methods of treatment can be used to try to improve the overall efficiency and functioning of the defence mechanisms of the body. These can include deep relaxation methods, various bodywork approaches, hydrotherapy, detoxification methods and others.

Finally, a number of safe techniques can be employed which ease symptoms and which aim to make life more comfortable.

There are many such methods including acupuncture, some forms of medication, bodywork methods and others.

In the next chapter we will take a closer look at myofascial trigger points, which are a major cause of pain in muscles and joints in FMS and in non-FMS patients alike. Whatever else is done to relieve FMS pain, attention to trigger points is an essential approach. Without an attempt to find and deactivate the trigger points which are creating pain symptoms, success will be slowed enormously. Dr. Lowe, who was mentioned earlier in relation to thyroid rehabilitation, is clear that in order to normalize the status of FMS patients, bodywork which pays attention to trigger points is an essential component (along with normalizing thyroid hormone function).

My own experience of treating a great many people with FMS and with myofascial pain symptoms is fully in agreement with Dr. Lowe's viewpoint, that trigger points need to be deactivated and the soft tissues and joints restored to functional normality, usually by a combination of treatment and self-care (stretching, exercise, etc.).

### Central sensitization

Scientists now describe the pain of fibromyalgia as involving increased sensitivity of the brain and central nervous system – known as central sensitization – where sensations that were previously mild are registered by the brain as being severe. Fortunately we now know that by reducing local sources of pain (for example in muscles, joints) central sensitization also reduces. (Affaitati *et al.*, 2011)

Sensitization can also be reduced by appropriate relaxation and breathing rehabilitation methods,

There is also evidence that trigger points contribute to the development of central sensitization (Niddam *et al.*, 2008).

# 4

# The Muscles and Fibromyalgia

### 'Normal' and abnormal muscle pain

What will be described in this chapter is the way in which normal muscles adapt to many different forms of stress, leading to the development of fibrosis and various forms of facilitation (hyper-irritability). While this is certainly a great part of what happens in fibromyalgia, other events are also taking place in the muscles that are a little different to this. At the end of the chapter, some ideas as to what is thought to be happening in fibromyalgia are discussed.

### How muscles react to stress

The muscles of the body respond to the stresses they are exposed to in an understandable sequence. We need to know about this sequence if we are to make sense of painful conditions such as fibromyalgia.

Muscles become more tense than they were in their relaxed state whenever they are asked to perform a function – to work, moving a part of the body, holding something in place or whatever, whether this is in our everyday life, our work or our sporting activities.

This increase in tension in the muscle when it prepares for, or carries out, an activity is described as the muscle developing increased 'tone'.

If these activities involving movement or the holding of a fixed position are repeated frequently, then the tone in the muscles can become more or less permanently increased.

The sort of demands that lead to increases in tone in muscles can be summarized as 'new use', overuse, misuse and abuse. Here are some examples:

- many muscles dramatically increase in tone in response to emotional stress
- specific muscles will increase in tone as a response to altered breathing patterns (see Chapter 2, Anxiety and/ or Hyperventilation and Fibromyalgia), which may be emotionally related or due to habit or to disease (asthma, bronchitis)
- muscles used in a repetitive way in sport, playing a musical instrument, performing a work function and so on will show an increase in tone, with some local areas of the muscle being more stressed than others
- the fascia of the body – the slightly elastic material that supports, divides, surrounds and gives shape and form to muscle (and which comprises one single, continuous web of material from the inside of the skull to the soles of the feet) – can be distorted, warped or stressed in numerous ways (for example, by injury to the skull due to forceps delivery, or because of in-born defects such as one leg being shorter than the other) and this will negatively affect and stress the muscles (increasing their tone) because they are so intimately bound up, literally, with the fascia (a simple example of what can happen is the fascial 'drag' that could occur in someone who has a dropped arch, as this would exert a pulling stress on the

fascia of the leg and, because of the continuity of the fascia, this would affect muscle structures all the way up to the back of the head)

- particular muscles will increase in tone when demands are made on them to stabilize or hold a posture in a sustained way (stooped, round-shouldered, military posture, sitting cross-legged and so on)
- if there are problems involving one leg being shorter than the other (most people have slight differences in leg length, but if the difference is more than 13 mm/ half an inch, the adaptation required can become a major mechanical stress factor) or if there is a tendency to hypermobility (looseness) in the joints, then muscles will be stressed and overworked as they compensate for slackness in the ligaments ('loose ligaments', an inborn feature, is commonly found in children with fibromyalgia)
- muscles will alter in tone if the joint they are associated with becomes restricted – through injury or arthritis, perhaps – just as sustained increase in muscle tone will cause joints to become restricted
- there are complicated reflex connections between the eyes and muscle tone, so, in many situations, the muscles of a part of the body will respond when the eyes move or are held in a particular direction, 'preparing' to move the body in that direction by increasing tone in the muscles that will perform that function. Therefore, eye imbalances, if not corrected by appropriate lenses and/ or prisms, can cause a constant amount of 'increased muscle tone' in certain muscles.

Regarding the last point, try the following for yourself.

With your eyes open, look upwards toward your forehead (with the eyes only, not by tilting your neck!). With your eyes rolled upward in this way, slowly bend forwards until you cannot easily bend any further.

Stop at this point and, without exerting any effort to bend yourself further, let your eyes move from looking upwards to looking down towards your chin. Now see how easily you can bend further towards the floor.

- When you were looking upwards, the tone of the muscles in your back increased (they were tensing), preventing you from bending forwards as far and as easily as when you were looking downwards.
- These eye reflexes are intimately connected with the position of various pelvic structures. If there are muscular or joint imbalances in the lower back or pelvis, this can affect the eyes and the eyes can further affect other muscles, as described above.

These are just some examples of reasons for muscle tone becoming greater – there are many more, including emotional factors.

When you are emotionally upset, angry, anxious or frightened, some specific muscles will tense and often remain tense for many hours until the emotion calms down (emotions usually affect the muscles in the shoulders and neck most strongly). If strong emotions are held not for hours but for years, the effects on muscles will be profound.

## WHEN INCREASED MUSCLE TONE BECOMES A PROBLEM

When a muscle is held in a state of increased tone – for any of the reasons given, or others – for more than a short time, three things happen.

1   The tension in the muscle causes it to require more oxygen, and this in turn demands increased blood flow to it. However, this demand for more oxygenated blood may not

be adequately met in all parts of the muscle because of the increased pressure on the blood vessels carrying the blood. This in its turn leads to an aching sensation, followed by pain if the oxygen does not arrive.

2   At the same time, the drainage away from the muscle(s) of waste products is slowed down by the increased muscle tone, leading to more aching.

3   The discomfort or pain resulting from inadequate oxygenation (known as ischemia or hypoxia) and the retained waste products leads to a further increase in tone, making matters worse. We now have a pain-increased tone-pain cycle.

4   To see just how quickly this happens, try the following. Sit back comfortably in a chair and raise one leg from the floor (or just clench your fist) and do nothing until the ache becomes unbearable. How long does the ache take to develop in your leg or arm? A few minutes only as a rule. Notice also what helps to get rid of the ache after you have had enough of holding one or other of these positions. Movement, a clenching and unclenching of the fist, or shaking the leg, or moving around on it gets the circulation and drainage back to normal. This is true in everyday life as well – movement and exercise that is not stressful will help to remedy the negative effects on muscles of static, non-moving stress positions. Now, imagine this sort of increased tone situation happening to many muscles, many times a day, for many months or years. What do you think would happen?

5   Over time, the muscle(s) would begin to adapt to the constant increased level of tone and the

circulatory changes by modifying their very
structure – elastic tissue start to develop more
solid areas; fibrosis starts to appear. As these
changes occur, patterns of chronic discomfort
begin and a lot of energy would be wasted.

## WHAT HAPPENS IF SUCH STRESSES BECOME CHRONIC?

When muscular stress becomes chronic – as a result of any combination
of emotional or postural or overuse or compensating (short leg and so
on) muscular stress factors, lasting not for minutes or hours but for
days or weeks or months or years – the soft tissues (muscles, tendons)
involved respond in quite predictable ways, as follows:

- The muscles themselves start to lose their elasticity and
  develop fibrous changes (just like the tough 'stringy' bits
  in an old chicken or a tough piece of beef or mutton) –
  just feel the tight bands in the muscles between your
  neck and shoulder to become familiar with fibrosis!
- What is happening is that, in response to a *functional*
  change – increased tone – there is an adaptive
  *structural* compensation.
- The muscles that have increased in tone, or tightness,
  will also be 'pulling' on their tendons, the structures that
  anchor them to bones, and the tendons themselves will
  be going through the same process of lack of oxygen,
  pain and sensitivity and, in time, they too will suffer
  fibrous change such as those the muscles went through.
  At the same time, the insertion point of the tendon into
  bone will become increasingly sensitive (called *periosteal
  pain points*).
- Any muscle held in a state of increased tone will
  be burning energy at a phenomenal rate – the
  musculoskeletal system is the greatest energy user of
  any of the body's systems and, if much of it is tense for a

great deal of the time, the amount of energy wasted will be profound. Any fatigue being felt by a person with such tense muscles, therefore, is not at all surprising.

- Because there is a direct relationship between the tone of a muscle and the relative 'weakness' in its directly opposite muscle, imbalances will start to develop, with one muscle group being tense and its antagonist(s) becoming weak. An example is that of very tight lower back muscles in someone who has very weak abdominal muscles.

- This process of one muscle (or group of muscles) influencing another is called *reciprocal inhibition* and it is this that allows you to gently lift and place a glass of water to your lips. The muscle contracting and bending your arm is allowed to perform this action smoothly only because its opposite number on the back of your arm is gently 'weakening' (relaxing) and allowing non-jerky movement to occur.

- If muscles become more or less permanently tense and fibrous, their opposite numbers will become more or less permanently weakened, leading to a degree of imbalance and lack of coordination in the performing of normal movements, causing unnatural and uneven wear and tear of the joints.

- This effect on the joints reflexively leads to further negative influences on the muscles which attach to, or are associated with, that joint.

- Some muscles – known as *postural muscles* because they are more involved in stabilizing and supporting the body than in moving parts of it – respond to the stresses described above differently to those muscles that have a more active, moving function (the so-called phasic muscles).

- This can best be summarized by saying that postural muscles shorten and phasic muscles weaken when they are stressed.
- If the changes described above take place, then structural changes in the person's short, tight postural muscles would be having a more or less constant effect on the function of the muscles themselves and on their antagonists (opposing muscles), as well as on the joints they support and move, which would in time become restricted and stiff.
- There would be imbalances – chronically stressed muscles, with their increased tone and increasing fibrosis, would be causing weakness in their antagonists while, at the same time, the tense muscles, if they are of a postural type, will become more or less permanently shortened, with joint stress also being a feature.
- In most people with chronic pain there are common and predictable chain reactions of shortness-weakness-shortness-weakness in postural muscles (see Figure 4.1) and there are multiple areas of sensitivity (Vladimir Janda, 1988, Gwendolen Jull and Vladimir Janda, 1987). These result from postures in which the muscles of the back of the leg, in particular, are tight and short, the lower back muscles become very tight, the belly is sagging, the shoulders are rounded, and the head is thrust forward of the body with the neck kinked forwards. Someone with these postural changes would not be able to breathe normally because of the crowding of the chest and the pressure on the diaphragm. Many of these postural changes will be only too familiar to anyone with fibromyalgia.

**Figure 4.1** *There is tightness in the pectoral, upper trapezius, levator scapula, scalene and sternomastoid muscles and weakness in the lower trapezius, middle trapezius and rhomboid muscles, producing what is called the 'upper crossed syndrome' in which joint stress, muscle pain and possible weakness, imbalance and breathing dysfunction all coexist.*

Pain is also usually a feature of all these general muscular changes involving tightness and weakness, but this sequence of negative soft tissue changes is only a part of the story because localized changes (the formation of trigger points) will have been taking place in the affected muscles at the same time that the general shortening and weakening changes were occurring. These are among the key features of fibromyalgia and, indeed, of most musculoskeletal pain problems.

## THE REFLEX PATTERNS AND FACILITATION

To facilitate is to 'make easy', to allow for something to happen more smoothly and easily than otherwise. In the body, when an area is stressed repetitively and chronically, the local nerve structures in that area tend to become overexcitable, more easily activated and hyper-irritable – this is called *facilitation*.

There are two very important forms of facilitation. If we are to make sense of muscle pain in general we have to understand these, so let us look at this more closely.

### Segmental facilitation

Our internal organs are supplied by nerves that leave the spine at specific levels. So, for example, the heart is supplied by nerves that leave the spine from the upper thoracic vertebrae, just below the base of the neck.

If, for whatever reason, the heart is, say, diseased or stressed, there will be feedback of impulses/messages along these same nerves towards the spine, and the muscles alongside the spine at that upper thoracic level will become tense. If the heart problem continues the area will become facilitated, with the nerves of the area, including those passing to the heart, becoming hyper-irritable.

If electrical readings of the muscles alongside the spine were taken they would show this upper thoracic region to be very active compared with the area above and below it. Also, the muscles alongside the spine at that level would be very tense and probably painful on pressure.

If something, anything, then caused 'stress' to the person who was affected in this way (say a loud noise or bad news or an argument or suddenly being caught in a cold downdraught of an air conditioner or absolutely anything that imposes stress on the person as a whole, not just this particular part of their body), there would be a dramatic increase in nerve activity in the facilitated area, but not in the rest of the spine.

The area would act in just the same way as a magnifying glass through which sunlight is shining, in that it would concentrate the nerve activity to a local fine point in the facilitated area, creating more nerve activity (and so stressing the heart more), and there would also be a local increase in muscle tension at that particular level of the spine.

Similar segmental (spinal) facilitation develops in response to any organ problem, obviously affecting only the part of the spine from which the nerves to that particular organ (liver, stomach, kidneys and so on) emerge. Other causes of segmental (spinal) facilitation can include stress imposed on a part of the spine through injury, overactivity, repetitive stress, poor posture or structural imbalance (one leg being shorter than the other, for example).

Whichever part of the spine is being chronically stressed (and the muscles alongside it) would become very tender indeed when pressed, and probably painful.

### Local (trigger point) facilitation in muscles

A similar sequence of events occurs when particularly easily stressed parts of muscle (where they insert into a bone, for example) are overused, abused, misused, disused in the ways discussed earlier in this chapter.

Localized areas of tension will develop in the muscle tissue, sometimes with a swollen feel, sometimes with a stringy or nodule-like feel, but always with a sensitivity to pressure. These local areas are easy to feel by palpating certain muscles. For example, most people have such areas in the muscle between the neck and shoulder (see Figure 4.2, page 93).

These palpably painful, tender, sensitive, localized facilitated points are called trigger points (or, more accurately, myofascial trigger points) because they are not only painful themselves when pressed, but when active will also transmit or activate pain sensations some distance away from themselves, in 'target' tissues.

Just like the facilitated areas alongside the spine, these 'points' will be made more active by stress of any type affecting the person in whom they are found, not just stress to the area in which they lie. When they are not actively sending pain to a distant area, producing symptoms which are recognisable to the patient, trigger points (local tender or pain areas) are said to be 'latent'.

**Figure 4.2** *Muscles such as the upper trapezius, scalenes and sternomastoid should be squeezed in a pincer-like hold rather than pressed because of sensitive structures underneath them. In this instance a trigger point is being compressed, producing pain in the target zone.*

### What causes the trigger point to develop?

Janet Travell and David Simons are the two physicians who, above all others, have helped our understanding of trigger points (see their book, *Myofascial Pain and Dysfunction: The trigger point manual*, 1983). Dr. Simons has described the evolution of a trigger as follows:

> In the core of the trigger lies a muscle spindle (these tiny reporting stations influence the length at which a muscle is held) which is in trouble for some reason (any of many forms of stress). Visualize a spindle like a strand of yarn in a knitted sweater . . . a metabolic crisis takes place which increases the temperature locally in the trigger point, shortens a minute part of the muscle (called a sarcomere) – like a snag in a sweater – and reduces the supply of oxygen and nutrients into the trigger point. During

this disturbed episode an influx of calcium occurs and the muscle spindle does not have enough energy to pump the calcium outside the cell where it belongs. Thus a vicious cycle is maintained and the muscle spindle can't seem to loosen up and the affected muscle can't relax.

Dr. Simons has tested this concept and found that, at the centre of the trigger points, there is indeed a lack of oxygen compared with that existing in the muscles surrounding it.

Research by the acknowledged world experts on pain, Professors P. Wall and R. Melzack (1989), has confirmed that while certainly not the cause of all pain, trigger-point activity is at least a part (often the major part) of almost all chronic pain situations and conditions.

Dr. Travell has confirmed that the following factors can all help to maintain and enhance trigger-point activity:

- nutritional deficiency, especially of vitamins C, the B complex and iron
- hormonal imbalances, such as low thyroid hormone production or function, menopausal or premenstrual situations
- infections, such as bacteria, viruses or yeast allergies – to wheat and dairy products in particular
- low oxygenation of tissues, aggravated by tension, stress, inactivity, poor breathing habits.

### Do trigger points actually cause fibromyalgia?

A condition called Myofascial Pain Syndrome (MPS) is a disorder in which pain of a persistent, aching type is referred to a target area from trigger points lying some distance away. Usually this is localized rather than general pain such as occurs in fibromyalgia.

---

This phenomenon has long been recognized as a cause of chronic pain in many people.

Many experts insist that the tender points palpated when assessing someone's condition when diagnosing fibromyalgia need to refer pain elsewhere if they are to be taken seriously in the diagnosis (making them trigger points by definition). The question needs to be asked – are myofascial pain syndrome and fibromyalgia the self-same thing? The answer, in short, is not quite.

Scandinavian researchers showed in 1986 that around 65 per cent of people with fibromyalgia had identifiable trigger points. It is clear, therefore, that there is an overlap between the two conditions.

Dr. P. Baldry, a leading British physician/acupuncturist, has summarized the similarities and differences between these two conditions in his book *Acupuncture: Trigger points and musculoskeletal pain* (1993).

The two conditions are similar or identical in that both fibromyalgia and myofascial pain syndrome:

- are made worse by cold weather
- may involve increased sympathetic nerve activity and conditions such as Raynaud's phenomenon (cold hands and feet)
- have tension headaches and paraesthesia (tingling sensations) as a major associated symptom
- are unaffected by anti-inflammatory painkilling medication, whether it is of the cortisone type or standard formulations
- involve chronic widespread pain.

However, fibromyalgia and myofascial pain syndrome are different in that:

- myofascial pain syndrome affects males and females equally, whereas fibromyalgia mainly affects females

- myofascial pain syndrome is usually local to an area such as the neck and shoulders or lower back and legs (although it can affect a number of parts of the body at the same time), whereas fibromyalgia is a generalized problem, often affecting all four 'corners' of the body at the same time
- muscles which contain areas that feel 'like a tight rubber band' are found in the muscles of around 30 per cent of people with myofascial pain syndrome, but more than 60 per cent of people with fibromyalgia
- people with fibromyalgia have poorer muscle endurance (the muscles get tired faster) than do the muscles of people with myofascial pain syndrome
- myofascial pain syndrome can sometimes be bad enough to cause disturbed sleep; in fibromyalgia, the sleep disturbance has a more causative role and is a pronounced feature of the condition
- myofascial pain syndrome produces no morning stiffness, whereas fibromyalgia does
- there is not usually fatigue associated with myofascial pain syndrome, while it is common in fibromyalgia
- myofascial pain syndrome can sometimes lead to depression (reactive) and anxiety, whereas, in a small percentage of fibromyalgia cases, some leading researchers believe that these conditions can be the trigger for the start of the condition
- conditions such as Irritable Bowel Syndrome, dysmenorrhoea (painful or difficult periods) and a feeling of swollen joints are noted in fibromyalgia but seldom in myofascial pain syndrome
- low-dosage tricyclic antidepressant drugs are helpful in dealing with the sleep problems and many of the symptoms of fibromyalgia, but not of myofascial pain syndrome

- exercise programmes (cardiovascular fitness) can help some fibromyalgia patients, according to experts, but this is not usually a helpful approach in myofascial pain syndrome
- the outlook for people with myofascial pain syndrome is excellent, as the trigger points usually respond quickly to therapeutic massage, manipulative or acupuncture techniques. The outlook for fibromyalgia is less positive, with a lengthy treatment and recovery phase being the norm unless specific causes can be identified (for example thyroid imbalance).

Trigger points are certainly part – in some cases the major part – of the pain suffered by people with fibromyalgia, and when they are (and they certainly are if pressure on the 'tender point' produces pain somewhere else in the body *which the patient recognizes as part of their pain pattern*) we need to know more about them and how they can be successfully treated.

## Summary of trigger point characteristics

- Dr. Janet Travell, a leading researcher into trigger points, defines them as being 'hyper-irritable foci lying within taut bands of muscle which are painful on compression and which refer pain or other symptoms at a distant site'.
- Embryonic (new) trigger points will develop as 'satellites' of existing triggers in the target area and, in time, these will produce their own satellites.
- According to Professor Melzack, nearly 80 per cent of trigger points are in exactly the same positions as known acupuncture points as used in traditional Chinese medicine.
- Painful points ('tender points') that do not refer symptoms to a distant site are simply latent triggers that need a little (or a lot) more stress to create greater facilitation and so turn them into active triggers.

- The taut band in which a trigger lies will twitch if a finger is run across it, and is tight but not fibrosed as it will soften and relax if the appropriate treatment is applied – something fibrotic tissue cannot do.
- Muscles that contain trigger points will often hurt when they are contracted (that is, when they are working).
- Trigger points are areas of increased energy consumption and lowered oxygen supply due to inadequate local circulation. They will therefore add to the drain on energy and the fatigue being experienced.
- The muscles in which trigger points lie cannot reach what is known as their 'normal resting length' – they are held almost constantly in a shortened position .Until the muscle housing a trigger point can reach this normal resting length without pain or effort, any treatment of the trigger point will only achieve temporary relief as they will reactivate after treatment.
- Stretching of the muscles using either active (patient stretches it) or passive (someone else stretches it) methods is a useful way of treating the shortness as well as the trigger point, because this can reduce the contraction (taut band) as well as increasing circulation to the area.
- There are many ways of treating trigger points, including acupuncture, Procaine injections, direct manual pressure (with the thumb and so on), stretching the muscle, ice therapy and others.
- Some of these methods (pressure, acupuncture) cause the release in the body and the brain of natural painkilling substances – endorphins – which explains one of the ways in which pain is reduced by such treatment. Pain is also relieved when one sensation (finger pressure, needle) is substituted for another (the original pain). In this

way pain messages are partially or totally blocked from reaching or being registered by the brain.

- Other treatment methods (stretching, for example) alter the circulatory imbalance affecting trigger points and, in this way, appear to deactivate them.
- The target area to which a trigger refers pain will be the same in everyone if the trigger point is in the same position, but this pattern of pain distribution does not relate to known nerve pathways or to acupuncture meridian pathways.
- The way in which a trigger point relays pain to a distant site is thought to involve one of a variety of neurological mechanisms, which probably involves the brain 'mislocating' pain messages it receives via several different pathways. The truth is that, as yet, we do not fully understand *how* trigger points produce their symptoms.
- The sites of trigger points lie in parts of muscles most prone to mechanical stress, producing circulatory inadequacy and lack of oxygen, among other changes.
- Trigger points become a self-perpetuating cycle (pain leading to increased tone, leading to more pain) and will never go away unless adequately treated.

### How reliable are palpation tests for tender and trigger points?

In 1992, a study was conducted by Frederick Wolfe, David Simons, *et al.*, to see how accurate palpation for tender points and trigger points was when used by experts who would be making the all-important diagnosis of fibromyalgia or myofascial pain syndrome. Volunteers from three groups were tested – some with fibromyalgia, some with myofascial pain syndrome, and some with no pain or any other symptoms.

The fibromyalgia patients were easily identified – 38 per cent of them were found to have trigger points. Of the myofascial pain syndrome patients, only 23.4 per cent were identified as having trigger points, and of the healthy volunteers, fewer than 2 per cent had any.

Incidentally, most of the myofascial pain syndrome patients had tender points in sites usually tested in fibromyalgia, and would have qualified for this diagnosis as well.

## What's going on in the fibromyalgia sufferer's muscles?

All of the adaptations and changes described above are likely to be taking place in the muscles of someone with fibromyalgia – plus a number of additional factors, which are as follows.

- A biochemical imbalance seems to be present, which may be the direct result of the negative effect of disturbed sleep, which leads to inadequate growth hormone production and, therefore, poor repair of minor muscle damage. There are also, commonly, low levels of a substance called serotonin in the blood and tissues. When serotonin is in low concentrations there are lowered pain thresholds (we feel pain more keenly), for two reasons: because of the reduced effectiveness of the body's natural endorphin painkillers, and because of the increased presence of something called 'substance P', which increases pain perception.

- The sympathetic nervous system – which, among other things is in control of the degree of muscle tone – can become disturbed, though research has not shown quite what form this takes. The disturbance can lead to muscle ischemia (lack of oxygen) beyond that experienced by 'normal' muscles, as described earlier in this chapter. This could lead to greater quantities of substance P being released and increased pain sensitivity.

- Some researchers propose that these two elements are combined in fibromyalgia, so that disordered sleep – leading to reduced serotonin levels, leading to reduced natural painkilling effects of endorphins – combines with a disturbed sympathetic nervous system to result in muscle ischemia and increased pain sensitivity. Both disturbances involve substance P being released, leading to reduced pain thresholds and activation of latent trigger points, with fibromyalgia as the end result.

- Some researchers propose that a great deal of 'micro-trauma' (tiny amounts of damage) of muscles occurs in fibromyalgia sufferers (for reasons that are not yet clear, but genetic predisposition is a possibility) , leading to calcium leakage in the tissues, which increases muscle contraction, further reducing oxygen supply. This micro-trauma seems also to be associated with a reduction in the muscle's ability to produce energy, so causing it to fatigue more easily and be unable to pump the excess calcium out of the cells. A similar mechanism is said by Travell and Simons to be involved in myofascial trigger point activity.

- James Daley, MD, has tested just what happens in the muscles of people with chronic fatigue syndrome (ME) when they exercise (Fibromyalgia Network Newsletter, 1990). A similar test involving people with fibromyalgia (by Robert Bennett, MD, Fibromyalgia Network Newsletter, 1990) gave similar results, which were that these people's muscles produced a great amount of lactic acid, which added to their discomfort. Some of the patients showed a dramatic rise in blood pressure during exercise; about a third had erratic breathing when exercising, and many also had low carbon dioxide levels when resting – which is an indication of a hyperventilation tendency (see Chapter 2). There is some evidence that progressive cardiovascular training (graduated training through exercise) improves muscle function and reduces pain in fibromyalgia, but this is not thought desirable (and is often quite impossible anyway because of the degree of fatigue) in chronic fatigue syndrome (ME).

## RESEARCH IMPLICATES RECTUS CAPITIS POSTERIOR MINOR (RCPM)

In Chapter 2 mention was made of the high incidence of FMS following whiplash injury. Possible explanations for this are suggested by a remarkable discovery made in 1994, when a dissection of a body at a dental school (University of Maryland, Baltimore) showed that a small muscle (Rectus capitis posterior minor – RCPM) which had long been thought to attach only to the base of the skull and the first bone of the neck, the atlas, actually had another connection altogether, to the lining of the spinal cord and brain, the dura, where it leaves the skull.

Further research has shown this muscle to be capable of producing severe pain when damaged in whiplash-type injuries, or when it is severely stressed (G. Hack *et al.*, 1995).

The function of this muscle, which was previously thought to be part of the control of head movement, was now seen actually to prevent the dura from folding on itself when the neck is kinked or the head thrust forwards ('chin poking').

Because of its position close to important circulatory centres, any dysfunction of this muscle has implications regarding circulation of blood and cerebrospinal fluid into and out of the head.

### Research shows whiplash can lead to FMS

As mentioned in Chapter 2, in 1997 Israeli researchers investigated over 100 patients with traumatic neck injury (whiplash) and compared their findings with approximately 60 patients with severe leg injuries (D. Buskila, L. Neumann, 1997).

Approximately 12 months after the original trauma all the patients were evaluated for the signs and symptoms of fibromyalgia syndrome.

The findings were that, 'Fibromyalgia prevalence in the neck injury group was 13 times greater than the leg fracture group.'

Over 21 per cent of the patients with neck injury (none of whom had chronic pain problems before the injury) developed fibromyalgia within months of their neck trauma, compared with only 1.7 per cent of the leg fracture patients.

This research, especially when combined with knowledge of the vital role of Rectus capitis posterior minor, provides a very real opening to understanding why FMS is so common after whiplash injuries.

During whiplash the small muscles at the base of the skull (such as RCPM) can have their nerve supply damaged ('denervation'). This loss of nerve supply leads to the death of the muscle (which shows on the scans as atrophy and fatty degeneration).

This is exactly what was identified by SPECT scans in the necks of patients with chronic pain conditions such as FMS.

Research at the Department of Osteopathic Medicine, Michigan State University, College of Osteopathic Medicine utilizing magnetic resonance imaging of both RCP major and minor, which was performed on six patients with chronic head and neck pain, as well as on five healthy individuals, produced remarkable findings (R. Hallgren, P. Greenman *et al.*, 1993, 1994).

- In those with chronic pain these muscles were shown to have developed fatty degeneration (atrophy) in which muscle tissue had been replaced by fatty deposits.
- This was not seen in the healthy subjects.
- The researchers suggest that the damage to the nerves in these injured muscles may cause increased facilitation (see notes on facilitation earlier this chapter) of nerve activity which is felt as pain (personal communication to the author, October 1997).

The findings in the whiplash study described above and in Chapter 2, and the MRI observations of Hallgren, Greenman and their colleagues regarding Rectus capitis posterior minor following trauma, suggest that damage to this part of the neck offers a possible explanation for the onset of FMS, in some patients. It also opens the possibility of treatment using manual methods (such as cranial manipulation and acupuncture) as being useful in such cases (see Chapter 9 for self-treatment of this area using gentle strain/counterstrain methods).

## Summary

- Some of the many causes of muscle pain have been identified, ranging from overuse through abuse and misuse, with facilitation and trigger point activity being common.
- The special features of fibromyalgia seem to involve a combination of circulatory and nerve imbalances, which make the stress-caused changes that take place in normal muscle even more pronounced and the symptoms more unpleasant.
- There are also apparently imbalances within the muscles of those with fibromyalgia, possibly involving excess calcium (which causes contraction of muscle fibres and, therefore, a lack of oxygen) and a deficiency in the ability to manufacture energy (which is made even worse by the lack of oxygen).
- Micro-trauma of the muscles, perhaps due to a congenital factor, seems more common in fibromyalgia, along with slower healing and recovery from local damage. The reasons for this are as yet unidentified, but probably involve low growth hormone production.
- The use of tender points to identify fibromyalgia seems an accurate approach, but there are bound to also be trigger points in most sufferers.

- Trigger points, when identified (in fibromyalgia and myofascial pain syndrome), should be treated in one or more of the ways described in Chapters 6 and 8.
- There are numerous interacting elements in both fibromyalgia and myofascial pain syndrome sufferers, and manual therapy, nutrition, stress reduction, breathing and postural reeducation, exercise (in some cases), acupuncture, non-specific immune system modulation (see Chapter 7 in particular) and medication (orthodox and herbal), among other things, can all be useful in encouraging recovery.
- The main differences between fibromyalgia and myofascial pain syndrome are that with fibromyalgia the pain is widespread and general, not localized; it affects females predominantly, rather than equal numbers of both sexes; and the primary causes of fibromyalgia remain unknown, whereas trauma (injury or repetitive minor injuries) seem to be the main immediate causes of myofascial pain syndrome.

## Tender and trigger points

Recent research evidence shows that trigger points contribute to the development of central sensitization, and that most of the tender point sites tested in diagnosis of fibromyalgia, are in fact active trigger points – possibly serving as generators of fibromyalgia pain. Deactivation of these may be useful in treatment of FMS (Ge *et al.*, 2010).

# 5

# The Brain and Fibromyalgia (and Chronic Fatigue Syndrome)

It is not too surprising, as many symptoms of fibromyalgia are brain related, that research has focused on this mysterious organ.

Memory lapses, 'foggy brain' (an inability to concentrate) and dyslexic episodes (an inability to recall simple words) are all part of many people's fibromyalgia (and of most people's chronic fatigue). Modern technology has now identified what may be happening in the brain with these conditions.

Among the abnormalities found so far in many people with fibromyalgia and chronic fatigue syndrome (ME) are reduced blood flow and energy production in key sites of the brain. While any such changes might themselves merely be symptoms of the syndrome, it is thought by many researchers that the most important imbalance in these conditions probably lies in the brain and central nervous system itself.

### Brain scan results
New technology for visualizing the brain in a non-invasive manner (SPECT, BEAM, PET) have advanced beyond the methods of early

MRI scanning techniques and allow very precise identification of areas, and types, of dysfunction within the brain.

As reported in Fibromyalgia Network Newsletters (May 1993 Compendium, July 1993, January 1994), various different approaches are being used to try to understand the mechanisms of fibromyalgia and chronic fatigue syndrome (ME).

Among the reports to date:

- PET research has shown that there is a far lower degree of activity in the frontal lobes of the brains of people with chronic fatigue syndrome (ME) than is the case in normal individuals or in depressed people, the latter showing some lowering of activity in these areas.
- Dr. Jay Goldstein, using SPECT technology, examined 33 patients with chronic fatigue syndrome, 15 of whom also met the criteria for fibromyalgia, and the scans showed marked reduction in blood flow to parts of the brain, especially among the fibromyalgia sufferers (Fibromyalgia Network Newsletters, 1993, 1994, *Journal for Action for ME*, 1994).
- James Mountz, MD, and Laurence Bradley, using SPECT, examined the cerebral blood flow of 10 fibromyalgia sufferers and found a decreased flow in the region of the caudate nuclei (right and left), which is involved in memory and concentration as well as pain-regulation functions (Fibromyalgia Network Newsletters, 1993, 1994, *Journal for Action for ME*, 1994).
- Similar results have been found in those with sympathetic reflex dystrophy, although the blood flow decrease was greater in those fibromyalgia sufferers who had higher pain scores.
- 100 fibromyalgia sufferers who experienced chronic headaches were examined by Dr. Thomas Romano using SPECT, and 97 of them were shown to have blood flow

imbalances involving reductions in flow to regions of the brain (Fibromyalgia Network Newsletters, 1993, 1994, *Journal for Action for ME*, 1994).

■ Other technologies used to evaluate brain function all confirm what SPECT has shown, that there is deficient circulation to parts of the brain.

## The hormone link

The pituitary gland lies near the centre of the brain. It is this tiny organ that produces growth hormone. It is also an integral part of what is called the *hypothalamic-pituitary-adrenal axis*.

Four of the numerous end results of an imbalance involving the pituitary gland and this axis that are relevant to fibromyalgia could be:

1 an increase in substance P, leading to more feelings of pain
2 a decrease in growth hormone production, leading to poor repair of damaged muscle fibres
3 altered thyroid function
4 a decrease in energy production, leading to greater fatigue.

As hormonal imbalances have been identified as being one part of the complex of causes of fibromyalgia and chronic fatigue syndrome (ME), it is not surprising that premenstrual problems (in 40 per cent of fibromyalgia sufferers according to general surveys, but with far higher numbers according to some research – see Chapter 3), endometriosis and thyroid disturbances (a high percentage of people with underactive thyroids have fibromyalgia – see also Chapters 2 and 3) are all too common in both groups of sufferers.

Dr. Muhammed Yunus sees the imbalance in fibromyalgia as being at least partially due to a neuroendocrine disorder. He points out that pain and other symptoms common to fibromyalgia are transmitted through the central nervous system by chemicals called neurotransmitters (chemicals that either increase or damp down nerve connections/messages) such as substance P, which enhances pain transmissions (1989).

At the other end of the spectrum are neurotransmitters that *reduce* sensations of pain, such as serotonin, as well as derivatives of serotonin, epinephrine and dopamine.

When there is an excess of substance P and a deficiency of serotonin, for example, you can see easily that pain will be felt excessively.

Research has shown that in fibromyalgia there is indeed an excess of substance P in the spinal fluid (three times normal levels) and also that levels of serotonin (see also the discussion of sleep disorders in Chapter 3) in the brain are very low. Epinephrine and dopamine are also in short supply, so pain thresholds are low and pain, once felt, is maintained for longer (Fibromyalgia Network Newsletters, 1993, 1994, *Journal for Action for ME*, 1994).

Is this imbalance a cause or a symptom? Is the circulatory (and therefore oxygen) deficit in the brain a cause or a symptom? These sorts of questions need to be asked over and over again as we try to understand the condition.

### The limbic system – key to the brain's role in fibromyalgia?

The area of the brain most affected by poor blood supply seems to involve what is known as the limbic system, which includes several brain structures including the amygdala, hippocampus and the hypothalamus.

The limbic system and the network of nerves influenced by it can be visualized as a computer processing a vast amount of information arriving from the body, such as nerve messages and hormonal influences.

The limbic system then modifies and integrates all this information with the experience and attitudes the person has acquired and selects appropriate responses designed to improve the function and survival potentials of the individual.

The limbic system strongly influences homeostasis – the self-regulating and normalizing functions of the body which determine how well or ill we become.

Through interacting mechanisms involving both the limbic and nervous systems, as well as the hormonal (endocrine) system – all of which have been shown by different researchers to be out of balance in many people with fibromyalgia and chronic fatigue syndrome (ME) – a wide range of bodily functions can be affected, including:

- the stability of body temperature
- mood
- appetite
- functioning of the sympathetic nervous system immune system efficiency
- the selection of adaptive responses to stress memory regulation
- many functions concerned with sleep
- control of hormonal balance as well as a number of thought processes, including our emotional and behavioural responses to pain.

At its simplest, then, the limbic system controls our degree of pain tolerance, as well as having a powerful effect on how the immune system functions.

Dr. Jay Goldstein (author of *Chronic Fatigue Syndrome: The limbic hypothesis*, 1993) believes that the limbic system, if it is not functioning normally, could be responsible for many of the symptoms seen in fibromyalgia and chronic fatigue syndrome (ME), including the 'brain fog' symptoms, depression, dizziness, tinnitus (ringing in the ears), intolerance of alcohol, nasal allergies, tendency to gain weight, sensitivity to chemical smells and specific foods, breathing irregularities and many of the other symptoms. He believes that the limbic system disturbance may itself be the result of cytokine production by viral agents, as well as cytokines produced during exercise (discussed further below).

In support of this theory, Dr. Ismael Mena, using SPECT methods, has shown that the blood flow through that part of the brain known as the cerebral cortex, already low in chronic fatigue syndrome sufferers, is *further* reduced during exercise, rather than increased, which would be the body's normal response to active exercise (*Journal for Action for ME*, 1994).

## IS THIS BRAIN FACILITATION?

If you recall the discussion of facilitation in Chapter 4, in which areas of the spine, or local trigger points, become hyper-reactive, you will recognize that what seems to happen to the limbic system is very much the same as the sequence of events that occurs in nerves in the process of facilitation. Remember, facilitation takes place when, for a variety of stress-related reasons, parts of the nervous system become hyper-reactive, producing myofascial trigger points and facilitated segments along the spine.

If this happens to part of the brain that controls vast areas of the nervous and immune system, you can imagine the devastating end results – and fibromyalgia could be one of these. It is worth restating here that among the factors which make facilitation more likely is a thyroid hormone deficiency (as well as deficiencies of certain vitamins such as B-complex). The interconnections which exist between different symptoms and causes is complex. Biochemical and emotional stress factors impact on the nervous system and the brain in so many ways that is not always possible to decide what is a cause and what is an effect.

## CAUSE OR EFFECT?

Before looking more closely at imbalances in the brain and their possible link to fibromyalgia, a short diversion may be helpful in helping to sift out 'cause' from 'effect'.

The ultimate effect in FMS is represented by the symptoms – the pain, fatigue and distress. These symptoms eventually become so burdensome that they start to cause other symptoms, such as depression. So symptoms can become causes.

As we have already seen in earlier chapters, at least three forms of 'cause' can easily be attributed to these symptoms:

1   allergies/intolerances which are capable of producing all of the symptoms listed in CFS (ME) and FMS
2   hyperventilation, which carries with it a list of symptoms even longer than that which attaches to FMS
3   thyroid imbalance, which can result in all the symptoms of FMS and CFS.

We can also identify a number of conditions which could produce some of the main symptoms of FMS, including myofascial pain syndrome, yeast overgrowth (Candida), depression and so on.

## WHICH IS THE CAUSE AND WHICH IS THE EFFECT?

Allergy, hyperventilation and thyroid imbalance can all be shown to result from other causes . . . which makes these conditions symptoms themselves.

- Allergy can be shown to sometimes be caused by sensitization to substances which are entering the bloodstream due to a damaged intestinal mucous membrane and/or because of a toxic liver condition which prevents appropriate deactivation of allergens in the bloodstream. Therefore, the allergy is itself a symptom caused by other factors.
- Hyperventilation can result from various causes, but the main reason is thought to be habit, related to a feeling of anxiety. One of the main *results* of hyperventilation, however, is a state of anxiety, and being anxious leads to more hyperventilation. Is anxiety a cause or a symptom

of hyperventilation; or is hyperventilation a symptom or a cause of anxiety? The answer is sometimes both. So which is cause and which is effect?

- Thyroid imbalance can be caused by radiation damage, nutritional imbalance, toxicity, allergy, drugs, etc. So it is itself a symptom, which causes other symptoms (such as FMS).

This short look at causes and effects should be kept in mind when causes are seen to result from brain changes.

What causes these brain changes should be the question, and how can we best correct the causes?

## What are the causes?

What could cause the brain, or a major part of it, to become hyper-reactive, sensitized, facilitated? Could it simply be because of inadequate oxygen/ blood supply?

Dr. Jay Goldstein believes that the limbic system in people with chronic fatigue syndrome and fibromyalgia 'isn't working right. It is too sensitive to certain stimuli; it doesn't filter them out properly (through a mechanism called sensory gating), and it doesn't process the inputs correctly either.' But why does this happen?

Goldstein believes that early childhood experience of major stress (physical, biochemical or psychological) can lead to a dramatic increase in cortisol (stress hormone) levels which can affect parts of the brain both physically and in the way it functions (R. Sapolsky, 1990, 1994). He suggests that immature neural structures have 'a natural plasticity' which allows environmental stresses to 'programme' them to over-react to stimuli which are threatening to the individual (J. Goldstein, 1996).

In this way variations in inborn (genetic) characteristics, as well as aspects of upbringing and early exposure to stress, combine to produce the patterns in which the individual responds to later stress in either an exaggerated or an insufficient way, compared to 'normal' reactions.

According to Goldstein, the infant brain can be influenced by 'many triggering agents in the predisposed individual' including viral infections, 'immunizations which deplete biogenic amines' (A. Gardier *et al.*, 1992), toxic chemicals, trauma to the head, difficulties in delivery, electromagnetic fields, sleep deprivation, general anaesthesia, and stress (whether mental, emotional or physical). To these potential influences on brain circulation and function might be added the effects of hyperventilation as discussed above, as well as allergic reactions.

This idea of a system which has been programmed to react inappropriately to stimuli will be examined further in the next chapter (see Allostasis).

## POST TRAUMATIC STRESS AND FIBROMYALGIA

It is possible that something similar could occur in adult life. Research has shown that over 20 per cent of people who have a diagnosis of Post Traumatic Stress Disorder display all the symptoms of fibromyalgia (M. Amir, 1997). Could the major emotional and physical causes of PTSD sometimes be sufficiently disruptive of normal function to leave the nervous system, brain and hormonal system malfunctioning just as in those traumatized early in life?

The theories as to just why the brain and central nervous system are functioning in an unbalanced way are numerous.

■ Some experts cite immune system disturbances, which are themselves a result of toxic overload and/or viral activity operating within a pattern of inborn tendencies and susceptibilities. They say that it seems as though the multiple stresses of life can cause the defence mechanisms of vulnerable people to become activated and, ultimately, overburdened, leading to chaotic responses instead of orderly ones.

- Other researchers have focused on the hormonal imbalances commonly found in fibromyalgia sufferers, or the nervous system's overexcitability.
- The latter is itself influenced by the hormonal neurotransmitters, which are themselves influenced by nutritional and/or toxic and/or infectious disturbances such as viruses, yeasts, parasites and bacteria, which cause undesirable chemicals to be produced, leading to even greater immune system stress as well as bowel dysfunction and associated poor nutrient absorption, resulting in multiple allergies and sensitivity reactions.
- Alternatively, there could be abnormal functional patterns such as hyperventilation, which can be caused by – or which can cause – profound anxiety, itself producing fatigue and sleep disturbances and the repercussions of these.
- Otherwise, the causes could stem from any of a number of factors, ranging from poor stress-coping abilities to nutritional imbalances (too little magnesium, calcium, zinc or chromium, or, perhaps, too much sugar) with the biochemical mayhem that this could cause.
- Another theory is that the constant bombardment of the central nervous system and brain by messages from neural reporting stations in stressed muscles and myofascial trigger points, caused by postural and habitual use imbalances, could be *overloading* the pain-tolerance thresholds.
- Others hold the view that the whole complex of symptoms can be seen to be the result of disturbed mental and emotional patterns manifesting in the physical body, making the problem one that is best treated by a psychiatrist.

- Alternatively, the whole problem could be caused by trauma or silicone implants or a tick bite or vaccination or electromagnetic disturbances or a state of depression, which is itself caused by all or any of the above!
- Or the cause(s) of fibromyalgia could involve something else altogether that is as yet undiscovered.

## THE REALITY

What we have in reality is an imbalance caused by potentially any or all of the factors listed above, or others, in any combination – leading to what we have seen as being the likely scenario of biochemical, neuro-humoral (nerves and hormones acting together) and functional (circulation and so on) factors impacting on the brain and central nervous system with devastating effects on the way we function – with sleep disturbances, anxiety, fatigue, pain, digestive and a host of other symptoms emerging.

What is absolutely critical as we move forward to a consideration of what treatments may be useful, is to hold on to several very important facts. In this way we can avoid the mistake of trying to treat everything in sight, and focus instead on doing what is most likely to help the body to help itself to recovery, which can be done by using a selection of non-specific ('constitutional') approaches as well as a medley of possible direct or local methods for dealing with the symptoms.

The 'facts' are that the homeostatic mechanisms can be assisted towards recovery if we:

- remove as many factors as possible that are negatively impacting the body/mind: stress reduction, adequate wholesome diet, rest and exercise; eliminate infectious yeasts, viruses, bacteria, parasites; replenish deficiencies, whether these be nutritional or hormonal; remove contacts with allergens; reduce excessive muscle tone via bodywork and stretching; normalize postural

and use imbalances (including breathing retraining) and
so on

- modulate immune and general repair functions
and develop increased hardiness by use of suitable
constitutional (that is, non-specific) methods,
including counselling, hydrotherapy, general bodywork,
detoxification methods, deep relaxation methods
- treat the symptoms by means of appropriate medication,
acupuncture and other symptom-orientated methods
(injections into trigger points, for example).

One such approach to treating symptoms described in Chapter 6
is the use of the herb *Ginkgo biloba* and/or co-enzyme Q10, both of
which have been shown to increase the efficiency of the circulation
to the brain.

In the next chapter we will consider the beginning of a rational
approach to this complex of causes and symptoms.

### "Pain is in the brain"

Functional MRI neuroimaging scans have been used to show that
there are brain responses to light-touch pressure in people with
fibromyalgia, that are not evident in people without fibromyalgia.
This represents evidence of central sensitization, and one of the
main tasks in rehabilitation from chronic pain is to reduce this – by
the methods outlined in this and other chapters (Pujol *et al.*, 2009).

# 6

# Treating Fibromyalgia – the Associated Conditions

*Please note that the self-help measures outlined below (stress reduction, breathing and relaxation methods, hydrotherapy and nutritional and detoxification strategies) are not meant to be undertaken in isolation from responsible, professional advice and care, but are suggested as useful tactics to enhance whatever kind of care you are receiving.*

In this chapter we will be looking specifically at some of the key conditions that commonly occur with fibromyalgia – notably allergies, anxiety (coupled with hyperventilation and sleep disorders and general stress states), chemical sensitivity, toxicity, candidiasis, premenstrual syndrome, Irritable Bowel Syndrome and viral infections.

At the present time there are no clear guidelines as to what is the best approach for treating fibromyalgia. There is certainly evidence (much of it based on research studies) of the varying degrees of usefulness and success of, among other methods, osteopathic and/or chiropractic manipulative treatment, various other forms of bodywork including massage therapy and NeuroMuscular Therapy

(NMT), electro-acupuncture, metabolic rehabilitation (such as thyroid replacement), nutritional approaches, cognitive therapy, injections into pain points (tender points, trigger points), herbal medicine and specific drugs. Some of these will be examined or reported on in Chapter 9.

If any of the methods listed above, or others, produce a reduction in the 'load' being coped with by our defence mechanisms, then it is likely that the self-healing processes will become more effective again and start to actually normalize imbalances, rather than simply struggle to keep things going.

### Understanding homeostasis – self-healing

It is absolutely vital for anyone afflicted with a chronic illness to hold on to the fact that their body is a self-healing mechanism. Just as broken bones mend and cuts usually heal, and most ill-health – from infections to digestive disturbances – goes away with or without treatment, in a healthy state, there must be a constant process for normalization and health promotion in operation. This is called *homeostasis*.

The homeostatic functions (which include the immune system) can become overwhelmed if too many demands are made of them because of, perhaps, any or all of a selection of negative impacts (see Figure 6.1). These could be nutritional deficiencies, accumulated toxic material (environmental pollution, either of food or in the air breathed, in medication, previous or current use of drugs and so on), emotional stress, recurrent or current infections, allergies, modified functional ability due to age or inborn factors or acquired habits involving poor posture, breathing imbalances and/or sleep disturbances and so on. If this happens, at a certain point in time the adaptive homeostatic mechanisms break down and illness – disease – appears. This situation is called *heterostasis* (based on the research work of the great Canadian scientist Hans Selye, as described in his book *The Stress of Life*, 1980).

## ALLOSTASIS

If homeostasis describes the body defending and repairing itself efficiently in response to challenges and stress, and heterostasis is the state of affairs when homeostasis is overwhelmed and treatment is needed, *allostasis* describes what is happening when the brain, nervous and hormonal systems over – or under-react to whatever is happening to the individual (because, it is suggested, of excessive levels of early stress of a sudden, violent or excessive nature).

- Allostasis is seen to involve the release by the body of excessive stress hormones – often involving 'an expectation that things will go badly' with a sense that little personal control is possible – a state of chronic anxiety, in other words.
- These abnormal and excessive (or deficient) allostatic responses are accompanied by a range of hormonal imbalances which can influence almost any part of the body or its functions (B. McEwan, 1994).
- Animal studies show that lesions in the parts of the brain commonly thought by Goldstein to be involved in this process result in depressed immune function (natural killer cells in particular), a feature of CFS (J. Goldstein, 1996).
- Dysfunction of this part of the brain also produces a reduction in growth hormone production, with major implications for tissue repair and of particular importance in FMS.
- A change in the behaviour of that part of the brain which controls temperature in the body (thermoregulatory set point) may also occur and could account for temperature intolerance common in people with FMS and CFS.
- Goldstein reports 'constantly' seeing just such abnormalities in CFS and FMS patients – and has gone into great detail to explain the link between the changes

affecting different brain regions as a result of this sequence of events, and many of the multiple symptoms experienced – including pain, sleep disorders, poor cold tolerance, etc.

Understanding allostasis (and homeostasis) helps us to see why treatment strategies have to be carefully chosen in FMS, and that 'whole body', constitutional approaches are more likely to produce benefit than focused interventions which may be 'wrongly' interpreted by the brain.

The body needs help, treatment, and this can take the form of:

- reducing the load impacting the body by taking away as many of the undesirable factors as possible – by avoiding allergens, improving posture and breathing, learning stress-coping tactics, improving diet, using supplements if called for, helping normalize sleep and the circulation, introducing a detoxification programme, dealing with infections and generally trying to keep the pressure off the defence mechanisms while they focus on current, chronic repair needs
- enhancing and improving the defence and repair processes by a variety of means, mainly non-specific (see Chapter 7)
- treating the symptoms – while making sure that we are doing nothing to add further to the burden being borne by the defence mechanisms.

Not all of the possible beneficial methods available need to be used, because once the load on the self-repair processes is reduced sufficiently, a degree of normal homeostatic function is automatically restored and self-healing begins again. This means that it is necessary to focus attention on what seem to be the likeliest and easiest targets (perhaps employing a team approach in which more than one therapist/therapy is used) to achieve this desirable end. In one person this may call for a change of diet and stress reduction; for another, enhancement of immune function via avoidance of allergens, use of hydrotherapy and reduction in symptoms using simple bodywork and exercise may be enough for them to turn the corner.

## OPTIONS

- restoration of competence of immune system, enhancing defence capabilities and supporting repair functions, with the objective of improving adaptation processes
- reduction of multiple interacting stressors impacting the individual – without creating new problems – 'easing the load'
- empowering the patient – helping achieve a sense of control via education, retraining and counselling
- treating symptoms – as long as this does no additional harm
- complementary or alternative healthcare, encouraging homeostasis
- choosing from integrated bodywork approaches (osteopathy, chiropractic, massage, physiotherapy), rehabilitation of posture and breathing, nutritional support/detoxification (diet, supplementation), stress-reduction methods, acupuncture, exercise, non-toxic antifungal, antiviral antibacterial, antiparasitic methods, probiotic use, homoeopathy and herbal medication, psychotherapy, non-specific 'constitutional' methods, including bodywork (massage), healing, deep relaxation, meditation, autogenics, fasting, counselling and psychotherapy, as well as standard medical attention.

The end result of the catalogue of stressors and the ultimate breakdown of adaptive capabilities is 'vertical ill-health', multiple symptoms, 'walking wounded' with symptoms such as chronic fatigue and muscular pain as key features.

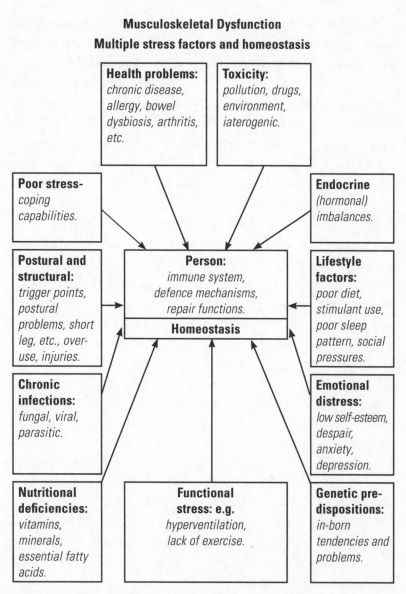

**Musculoskeletal Dysfunction**
**Multiple stress factors and homeostasis**

**Health problems:** *chronic disease, allergy, bowel dysbiosis, arthritis, etc.*

**Toxicity:** *pollution, drugs, environment, iaterogenic.*

**Poor stress-** *coping capabilities.*

**Endocrine** *(hormonal) imbalances.*

**Postural and structural:** *trigger points, postural problems, short leg, etc., over-use, injuries.*

**Person:** *immune system, defence mechanisms, repair functions.*

**Homeostasis**

**Lifestyle factors:** *poor diet, stimulant use, poor sleep pattern, social pressures.*

**Chronic infections:** *fungal, viral, parasitic.*

**Emotional distress:** *low self-esteem, despair, anxiety, depression.*

**Nutritional deficiencies:** *vitamins, minerals, essential fatty acids.*

**Functional stress: e.g.** *hyperventilation, lack of exercise.*

**Genetic pre-dispositions:** *in-born tendencies and problems.*

**Figure 6.1** *The body's homeostatic mechanisms, which defend and protect us, can be overwhelmed by a wide range of stress factors, leading to a state of ill health. At this stage, treatment is required to improve the defence capabilities and so restore homeostasis and/or ease the load of stress factors making demands on the body.*

**Non-specific approaches such as relaxation, massage and forms of hydrotherapy are often more beneficial than specific treatments, which make excessive adaptation demands.**

In this chapter, our focus is on describing the removal or modification of factors that may be negatively influencing the body/mind in people with chronic fatigue syndrome (ME) or fibromyalgia, starting with the major associated symptoms listed in Chapter 2. Some of the topics in that listing contain comments regarding treatment and so, to avoid repetition, they will not be covered again in this chapter.

In the next chapter we will be looking at what can best be called 'constitutional approaches' to health in general and the treatment of chronic fatigue syndrome (ME) and fibromyalgia in particular. In Chapter 8 our attention will be specifically on bodywork methods and self-treatments. In Chapter 9 our focus will be on research evidence as to 'what works' in treating fibromyalgia and its associated conditions.

## Allergies

Expert advice and guidance is needed in dealing with allergies, which are common in fibromyalgia and chronic fatigue syndrome (ME). Many tests exist, but none of them is foolproof and many have a tendency to produce false positive and false negative results. The most accurate method is to test suspected foods by eliminating them (for at least five days), seeing if there is a reduction in symptoms (or not) and then reintroducing the food and reassessing the symptom patterns. By completing the questionnaire in Chapter 2 (page 25) it should be possible to assess whether allergy/sensitivity is possibly a factor in your condition. Use of the 'pulse test' (below) offers another option, in which 'culprit' food and drinks can be identified. Even more accurate is elimination, where symptoms are evaluated when particular foods, or whole food families, are eliminated. If a challenge is then initiated, and the food is introduced again, and symptoms return, a clear indication is available as to the best course of action.

## PULSE TEST

- A simple pulse test is sometimes an accurate guide to food sensitivity.
- The pulse is taken before eating a particular food and then again at intervals after it has been eaten – 20 minutes, 40, 60 and perhaps 120 minutes.
- If the pulse rate changes by at least 10 beats per minute, either upwards or downwards, the food is suspect and should be avoided for at least a week before being retested.
- If the food is indeed provoking an allergic reaction, then if it is eaten twice on a single day, following a week's exclusion, the pulse rate should rise or fall by at least 10 beats per minute some time after (sometimes immediately) a meal containing the suspect food, and symptoms should appear.
- The food should then be eliminated from the diet for at least six months.

## EXCLUSION AND ROTATION DIETS

In general, food allergy is dealt with by eliminating the allergen(s) through specific exclusion or hypoallergenic diets – such as a lamb and pear diet or a monodiet of, say, rice only or a Stone Age dietary pattern, which eliminates all grains and dairy produce as well as modern, processed foods, or by short-term fasting (usually five days), followed by the reintroduction of suspected foods to assess their impact on symptoms. See details below.

Alternative methods include rotation diets, in which suspected foods are eaten infrequently (no more than once in five days) to avoid sensitization or allergic responses. The various methods currently in use by clinical ecologists or allergy specialists all require patience, conscious, dedicated application and sound advice to be effective. Stress reduction is also vital in dealing with allergy/sensitivity problems.

If bowel malabsorption problems exist, resulting perhaps from yeast or parasite activity, then the bowel condition needs to be sorted out concurrently with or before the allergy is tackled (see Candida and Irritable Bowel Syndrome, below).

Sometimes an allergy occurs when food is digested incompletely because inadequate levels of hydrochloric acid are produced or there is poor digestive enzyme production. Expert nutritional help can assist in normalizing such imbalances.

Various homoeopathic desensitization approaches are also found to be useful at times. Again, they should only be undertaken with expert guidance.

## Questionnaire: Identifying food intolerances ?

The identification of foods to which we are allergic or intolerant can be difficult. In some cases it is obvious, and we therefore avoid the food; in other cases we may need to undertake long and difficult detective work in order to identify culprits.

Make notes of the answers to the following questions

1 List any foods or drinks that you know disagree with you, or which produce allergic reactions (skin blotches, palpitations, feelings of exhaustion, agitation, or other symptoms).
NOTES

2 List any food or beverage that you eat or drink at least once every day.
NOTES

3 List any foods or drinks that, if you were unable to obtain them, would make you feel really deprived. ('What food would you miss most?')
NOTES


4 List any foods that you sometimes have a strong craving for.
NOTES


5 What sort of food or drink is it that you use for snacks? List these.
NOTES


6 Are there foods which you have begun to eat (or drink) more of recently?
NOTES


7 Read the following list of foods and underline twice any that you eat at least every day, and underline once those that you eat three or more times a week:

- Bread (and other wheat products); milk; potato; tomato; fish; cane sugar or its products; breakfast food; sausages or preserved meat; cheese; coffee; rice; pork; peanuts; corn or its products; margarine; beetroot; tea; yogurt; soya products; beef; chicken; alcoholic drinks; cake; biscuits; oranges or other citrus fruits; eggs; chocolate; lamb; artificial sweeteners; soft drinks; pasta.

When it comes to testing by 'exclusion', the foods that appear most often on your list (in questions 1 to 6 and the ones you've underlined twice) are the ones to test first – one by one.

- Decide which foods on your list are the ones you eat most often (say, bread), and test wheat and other grains (barley, rye, oats and millet) by excluding these from your diet for at least three weeks.
- You may not feel any benefit from this exclusion (if wheat or other grains have been causing allergic reactions) for at least a week. You may even feel worse for that first week (this is caused by withdrawal symptoms).
- If after a week your symptoms (fatigue, palpitations, skin reactions, breathing difficulty, muscle or joint ache, feelings of agitation – or whatever) are feeling better, you should maintain the exclusion for several weeks more before reintroducing the excluded foods – to challenge your body – to see whether symptoms return.
- If they do return after eating the foods, you will have shown that your body is better, for the time being at least, without the food you have identified.
- Remove these foods from your diet (in this case, grains – or wheat if that is the only grain you tested) for at least six months before testing it again. By then you may have become desensitized to it and be able to tolerate it again.
- If nothing was proved by the wheat/ grain exclusion, similar elimination periods on a diet free of dairy produce, or fish, or citrus, or soya products, etc. can also be attempted – using your questionnaire results to guide you – always choosing the next most frequently listed food (or food family).

This method is often effective. Dairy products, for example, are among the most common allergens in asthma and hay fever problems.

A range of gluten-free and dairy-free foods are now available from health stores, which makes such elimination far easier.

### Rotation diet and reaction diary (symptom score sheet)

There are other ways of reducing the stress of irritant foods which cause you symptoms, and one of these involves the use of a rotation diet, in which foods from any particular family of suspect foods (identified by the questionnaire, page 126) are eaten only once every five days or so.

This system is effective, especially if a detailed 'food and symptom diary' is kept, in which all deviations from your normal state of health are noted down, as are all foods eaten.

Symptoms such as feelings of unusual fatigue, irritability, difficulty concentrating, muscular pains or actual breathing difficulties should be listed and given a daily 'score' out of (say) 10, where 0 = no problems and 10 = the worst it has ever been.

Make sure to score each symptom each day to see how it varies, and to link this to when suspect foods are eaten (sometimes reaction to foods takes up to 12 hours to be noticed).

If such a score sheet is kept and note is made of suspect foods, a link may be uncovered.

By comparing the two lists (suspect foods and symptoms) it is often possible to note a pattern connecting particular foods and symptoms, at which time the exclusion diet described above can be started.

Another way of 'unmasking' allergy provoking foods is the 'Oligoantigenic diet'.

## OLIGOANTIGENIC DIET

The Oligoantigenic diet was developed at Great Ormond Street Hospital for Sick Children, London and at Addenbrookes Hospital, Cambridge as a means of identifying foods which might be causing or aggravating the conditions of young patients.

By avoiding foods which may be provoking symptoms for no fewer than five days, all traces of any of the food will have cleared the system and any symptoms caused by these should have vanished.

Symptoms which remain are either caused by something else altogether (infection, for example, or hormonal imbalance or emotions) or by other foods or substances.

On reintroduction of foods in a carefully controlled sequence (the 'challenge'), symptoms that reappear are shown to derive from a reaction to particular foods which are then eliminated from the diet for at least six months.

There is some evidence to support the idea that those foods which have become a major part of the human diet since Stone-age times – mainly grains (particularly wheat) of all sorts and dairy produce –are the most likely to provoke reactions.

All modern processed foods involving any chemicals, colourings, flavourings, etc. are also suspect.

The Oligoantigenic diet is usually followed for three weeks while a careful check is kept on symptoms (pain, stiffness, mobility, etc.). If symptoms improve or vanish, then one or more of the foods being avoided may be to blame.

Identification and subsequent avoidance of the culprit food(s) depends upon whether symptoms return when the food(s) are reintroduced.

The eating schedule listed below is a modified version of the hospital pattern. To try a modified Oligoantigenic exclusion diet, evaluate the effect of following a pattern of eating in which the foods as listed below are excluded for three weeks.

|  | **Allowed** | **Forbidden** |
|---|---|---|
| **Fish** | White fish, oily fish | All smoked fish |
| **Vegetables** | All | None, but people with bowel problems are asked to avoid beans, lentils, and cabbage, and to eat all vegetables cooked-Brussels sprouts |
| **Fruit** | Bananas, passion fruit, peeled pears, pomegranates, paw-paw (papaya), mango | All other fruits |
| **Cereals** | Rice, sago, millet, buck-wheat, quinoa | Wheat, oats, rye, barley, corn |
| **Oils** | Sunflower, safflower, linseed, olive | Corn, soya, 'vegetable', nut (especially peanut) |
| **Dairy** | None | Cow's milk and all its products including yogurt, butter, most margarine, cheese of all sorts, all goat, sheep and soya milk products, eggs |
| **Drinks** | Herbal teas such as camomile and peppermint | Tea, coffee, fruit squashes, citrus drinks, apple juice, alcohol, tap water, carbonated drinks |
| **Miscellaneous** | Sea salt | All yeast products, chocolate, preservatives, all food additives, herbs, spices, honey, sugar of any sort |

If benefits are felt after this three-week exclusion, a gradual introduction is made of one food at a time, leaving at least four days between each reintroduction. This will allow you to identify those foods which should be left out altogether – if symptoms reappear when they are reintroduced.

If a reaction occurs (symptoms return, after having eased or vanished during the three-week exclusion trial), the offending food is eliminated for at least six months and a five-day period of no further experimentation (reintroduction of previously excluded foods) is followed (to clear the body of all traces of the offending food).

After the five days, testing (challenge) can start again, one food at a time, involving anything you have previously been eating which was eliminated by the Oligoantigenic diet.

## CAUTIONARY NOTE

When a food to which you are strongly allergic and which you have been consuming regularly is stopped, you may experience 'withdrawal' symptoms for a week or so, including flu-like symptoms and marked mood-swings, anxiety, restlessness , etc. This will pass after a few days.

These 'withdrawal' symptoms can be a strong indication that whatever you have eliminated from the diet is responsible for a 'masked' allergy, which may be producing many of your symptoms.

### Anxiety, sleep disturbance and hyperventilation

In the simplest terms, the more anxious you are, the more easily aroused you will be and, as increased arousal stimulates the sympathetic nervous system, the more easily upset, tense and fatigued you will become because sleep will be disturbed.

The less anxious you are, the less aroused you will be, the less dominant your sympathetic nervous system will be and the less likely it is that sleep disturbance, and all that flows from that, will occur.

## Measuring arousal – an anxiety questionnaire **?**

There are a number of ways of assessing your arousal, including measurement of the electrical resistance of your skin, the amount of activity in key muscles when you are resting, and the type of brain wave activity most common in your brain. You can easily recognize that your arousal levels are high, at this time, as you will develop one or more of the signs pinpointed by the following questions:

- Are you more restless and/or easily upset than usual?

- Do you have difficulty relaxing?

- Has your sleep pattern been disturbed lately?

- Do you find yourself sighing a lot or breathing more shallowly than usual?

- Are you having difficulty concentrating?

- Do you feel 'on edge' much of the time?

- Are you conscious of an almost constant state of anxiety?

If you answered YES to more than one of these questions, then anxiety (and possibly hyperventilation) may be part of your condition. If so, there are strategies you can adopt to help yourself, and you might also consider getting professional help in acquiring stress coping methods and/or breathing retraining.

### WHAT'S TO BE DONE?
The solution is simple. You need to look at your lifestyle and decide whether or not your stress-coping abilities are adequate to the demands placed on them.

You need to consider the following:

---

- To be really relaxed and able to cope with stress, your diet needs to meet your requirements while your intake of 'tasty toxins' and stimulants (especially caffeine, alcohol and tobacco) needs to be as low as possible – zero, ideally.
- To be relaxed, the muscles need to release their tensions, leading to a saving of otherwise wasted energy. This might be achieved by massage, stretching, exercise, hydrotherapy (see Neutral Bath, described below) or better nutrition. Muscular release is the first step towards calming the mind (the mind cannot be calm if the muscles are in a state of tension), so use the breathing method, the autogenic training methods and the hydrotherapy technique described in this chapter, and the stretching and other techniques described in Chapter 8 to achieve this.
- To be relaxed, your breathing needs to be full and free. The exercises given below can be useful in achieving this, if the structural and mechanical tensions in your breathing apparatus are not too great. Bodywork treatment and stretching movements are almost certainly needed if the problems are chronic. It is hard to retrain breathing if the machinery which breathes is stiff and tight!
- Improved breathing leads to better circulation and oxygenation, and has specific effects on reducing feelings of anxiety and being stressed out. The body and mind cannot relax or cope well with stress if the brain is poorly supplied with oxygen and nutrients because of a poor blood supply.
- To be relaxed, once you have achieved muscular release and your breathing is no longer restricted, your mind needs to be able to stay still and focused and release itself from the chatter of daily events and anxieties. This leads to a profound sense of being centred and at ease – and those around you will notice as your ability to concentrate and remember details improves and you start to radiate calm instead of anxiety.

To summarize – muscular release, unrestricted breathing, mental calm. These three simple steps, undertaken in this sequence, can protect you from the worst effects of stress, as well as allowing you to feel, breathe and function better, reducing sympathetic overarousal.

Regarding breathing, you can start by learning a simple, traditional yoga breathing method which has been shown in medical studies to lower arousal/anxiety states very quickly indeed. Everyone who suffers from anxiety or stress should learn this!

To enter a state of relaxation you can also use one of a great many methods of relaxation, including autogenic training and hydrotherapy (described below).

## ANTI-AROUSAL BREATHING TECHNIQUE

Have you completed the Hyperventilation Questionnaire in Chapter 2 (page 31)? If it indicates over-breathing habits, and if the Anxiety Questionnaire, page 133, suggests that you need to be calmer, then the exercises below should help.

Before doing the exercise described below, sit or stand in front of a mirror and observe your shoulders as you breathe deeply. Do they rise towards your ears as you inhale?

If so, you are using certain muscles that attach to the neck and shoulders as well as the upper ribs in a way that should only happen when you are, or have been, running. To use them in this way when seated or standing shows they are overworking, and this will influence your breathing mechanics in a negative way.

To start to retrain yourself to stop this habit – which is all it is – and help reduce the tendency it produces towards hyperventilation/anxiety, do the following exercise.

### Preparation

1   Sit in a chair that has arms, and rest your arms on them.
2   As you practise deep breathing, make sure your elbows
    are firmly pressed downwards towards the floor, so that
    they are against the arms of the chair all the time. This is

because when you are pressing down with the elbows it is impossible to use the neck and shoulder muscles while you are breathing, which you were previously doing, and so you are obliged to use the correct breathing muscles (use this tactic at the same time as the rhythmic pranayama breathing described below or at any other time until you can sit in front of a mirror and inhale without your shoulders lifting towards your ears).

Also, as you breathe in the way described below, ensure that your abdomen moves outwards at the start of inhalation – this guarantees that the diaphragm is working normally – and flattens at the end of the breath.

## PRANAYAMA BREATHING

There are many exercises to help improve breathing, but there is just one that has been shown in medical studies to effectively reduce arousal and anxiety levels (*Journal of the Royal Society of Medicine*, 1981). This exercise is based on traditional yogic breathing. Follow the steps below.

1  Having placed yourself in a comfortable position (ideally seated as described under 'Preparation', above), inhale through your nose only while counting slowly to yourself up to two or three. (Doing this, you fill your lungs fairly quickly, having ensured that the diaphragm is moving adequately so that the stomach pushes outwards on inhalation and flattens on exhalation. The counting is necessary because the timing of the inhalation and exhalation phases of breathing are central to this exercise.)

2  Without pausing to hold the breath at all, exhale slowly through your mouth with your lips pursed (as when kissing), to a count of four, five or even six.(Count to yourself at the same speed as when you inhaled. It is most important that the breathing out is slow and continuous.

It is no use breathing the air out in the first two counts and then simply waiting until the count reaches five or six before inhaling again.)

3   Repeat the inhalation (to a count of two or three, as before) and then exhale slowly (the objective is that, in time, with practice, you should make the exhalation phase last a count of eight).

4   Repeat the cycles of inhalation/exhalation for several minutes, with at least six cycles per minute (each cycle should eventually last ten seconds – two in, eight out, although at first you may find two in, three or four out is all you can manage).

By the time you have completed ten or so cycles, your sense of anxiety should be much reduced and your awareness of pain lessened. Do this exercise for a few minutes every hour if you are anxious or whenever stress seems to be increasing.

## CONTROLLED PAUSE METHOD (TO IMPROVE $CO_2$ TOLERANCE)

The short 'test' mentioned in question 3 of the Hyperventilation Questionnaire in Chapter 2 (page 31) is based on the Russian Buteyko retraining method.

When you breathe out and hold the breath out, after a number of seconds you have a feeling of a need to breathe in again.

This is not because you need oxygen (there is more than enough of this in your body) but is because levels of $CO_2$ are building up, and triggering the feeling that you need to breathe again.

A 'normal' pause of this sort should be around 30 seconds, although 20 is seen as a common average.

If you feel an urge to breathe before 20 seconds, your $CO_2$ tolerance is low.

After doing the test you will have an idea of your present tolerance to $CO_2$.

The way to increase this is simply to practise the 'controlled pause' as often as you can remember . . . and no fewer than three times a day.

Remember to breathe again just as soon as the urge becomes apparent to you. Never hold your breath out by will-power.

Within a week or so of repeating this pause a number of times a day you will find that the amount of time you feel comfortable holding your breath out will increase, and after three or four weeks you should reach 20 seconds easily without strain.

This will then have the exact opposite effect of hyperventilation. It will calm you, and allow improved circulation as the smooth muscles around the blood vessels relax.

Pain levels should also drop as the changes occur which reverse the hyperventilation tendency.

## RELAXATION TECHNIQUE (MODIFIED AUTOGENIC TRAINING)

There are a vast number of relaxation exercises, but one in particular is a good one for you to use in self-treatment. Autogenic training is best learned from a fully trained instructor, but the following modified exercise is an excellent way of achieving some degree of control over muscle tone and/or circulation and, therefore, over pain. Do this exercise (Chaitow, 1992) every day, ideally twice a day, for ten minutes at a time.

1   Lie on the floor or in bed in a comfortable position, with a small cushion under your head if this is more comfortable, your knees bent if this is better for your back, your eyes closed. Do the breathing exercise described in 'Pranayama Breathing' for five cycles (one cycle equals an inhalation and an exhalation). Let your breathing resume its normal rhythm.

2   When you feel calm and still, focus your attention on your right hand/arm and say silently to yourself 'My right arm (or hand) feels *heavy*.' Try to imagine and feel your arm relaxed

and heavy, its weight sinking into the surface it is resting on. Feel its weight. Over a period of about a minute, repeat the sentence several times and try to stay focused on the weight and heaviness of the hand/arm. You will almost certainly lose focus, as your attention will wander from time to time. This is part of the training element of the exercise, to stay focused, so don't feel angry, just go back to focusing on the arm and its heaviness. You may or may not be able to sense the heaviness – it doesn't matter too much at first. If you do, stay with it and enjoy the sense of release, of letting go, that comes with it.

3 Next, focus on your left hand/arm and do exactly the same as you did for your right one for about a minute.

4 Now do the same for your *left* leg and then your right leg, for about a minute each, with the same message and focused attention.

5 Go back to your right hand/ arm, and this time say to yourself 'My hand is feeling warm (or hot).'

6 After a minute or so, do the same for your left hand/arm, then your left leg and then finally the right leg, each time saying the sentence about feeling warm and focusing your attention on it. If you actually feel warmth, stay with that sensation for a while and feel it spread. Enjoy it.

7 Finally, focus on your forehead and affirm that it feels cool and refreshed. Stay with this cool and calm thought for a minute before getting up.

By repeating the whole exercise at least once a day (10 to 15 minutes is all it will take), you will gradually find that you can stay focused on each region and sensation.

'Heaviness' is what you feel when your muscles relax, and 'warmth' is what you feel when your circulation to an area is increased, while 'coolness' is the opposite, a reduction in circulation for a short while, which is usually followed by an increase, due to the overall relaxation of the muscles.

Measurable changes occur in circulation and temperature in the regions being focused on during these training sessions, and the benefits of this technique to people with Raynaud's phenomenon and to anyone with pain problems has been proven by the results of years of research. It does require persistence, though, to experience these benefits. The exercise should be done daily for at least six weeks before benefits will be noticed. The most notable of these will be a sense of relaxation and better sleep.

## RELAXATION TECHNIQUE: PROGRESSIVE MUSCULAR RELAXATION (PMR)

1    Wearing loose clothing, lie with your arms and legs outstretched.
2    Clench one fist. Hold for 10 seconds.
3    Release your fist, relax for 10 to 20 seconds, and then repeat exactly as before.
4    Do the same with the other hand (twice).
5    Draw the toes of one foot towards the knee. Hold for 10 seconds. Relax. Repeat, and then do the same with the other foot.
6    Perform the same sequence in five other sites (one side of your body and then the other, making 10 more muscles) such as:
     — back of the lower legs – point and tense your toes downwards – and then relax
     — upper leg – pull your kneecap towards your hip – and then relax
     — buttocks – squeeze together and then relax
     — back of the shoulders – draw the shoulder blades together and then relax
     — abdominal area – pull in or push out the abdomen strongly and then relax
     — arms and shoulders – draw the upper arm into your shoulder and then relax
     — neck area – push your neck down towards the floor and then relax
     — face – tighten and contract the muscles around your eyes and mouth, or frown strongly and then relax.

7   After one week, combine muscle groups:
    —   hands/ arms on both sides – tense and then relax together
    —   face and neck – tense and relax all the muscles at the
        same time
    —   chest, shoulders and back – tense and relax all the
        muscles at the same time
    —   pelvic area – tense and relax all the muscles at the
        same time
    —   legs and feet – tense and relax all the muscles at the
        same time.
8   After another week, abandon the 'tightening up' part of
    the exercise
    —   simply lie and focus on different regions, noting whether
        they are tense. Instruct them to relax if they are.
9   Do the exercise daily.

**Research study compares autogenic training and PMR in fibromyalgia**
Italian researchers compared the benefits of autogenic training
(AT) and PMR (called Erickson's technique) for patients with
fibromyalgia (V. Rucco *et al.*, 1995).

They found that both groups benefited in terms of pain relief
if they carried out the exercise regularly, but that because PMR
is easier and quicker to learn, patients are more likely to perform
this regularly compared with AT.

Those learning AT complained of 'too many intrusive thoughts',
which is precisely what AT is designed eventually to quieten –
that's the 'training' part of the exercise.

HYDROTHERAPY: A NEUTRAL RELAXATION BATH
By placing yourself in a neutral bath – that is, one where your body
temperature is the same as that of the water – a profoundly relaxing
influence on the nervous system occurs. Interestingly, this method
was used to calm violent and disturbed patients in mental asylums
before tranquillizers appeared!

This is helpful in all cases of anxiety, when you feel stressed and for relieving chronic pain and/or insomnia. It is also ideal for reducing excessive fluid retention and is a general tonic for the heart.

A neutral bath should not be used if you have a skin condition that reacts badly to water or if there is serious cardiac disease (it may help, but get professional advice before trying it).

### Preparation

Fill your bath with water as close to 97°F (36.1°C) as possible, but no hotter (measure the temperature with a thermometer). The beneficial effects of a neutral bath occur when the water is at or very close to body temperature. Immersion in water at this neutral temperature has a profoundly relaxing, sedating effect and a calming influence on the activity of the nervous system.

### Method

1  Get into the bath and, if possible, have the water cover your shoulders, with a towel or sponge to support your head.
2  Stay in the bath for anything from 30 minutes to 4 hours. The longer you can stay in the water the better as far as relaxation effects are concerned. Keep the thermometer in the bath and check it every now and again during this time to ensure that the temperature does not drop below 92°F (33.3°C). It can be topped up periodically, but do not let the temperature go above 97°F (36.1°C).
3  After the bath, pat yourself dry quickly and get into bed for at least an hour.

AROMATHERAPY FOR STRESS REDUCTION AND BETTER SLEEP
The selection of oils described below have proven healing properties
– *none is meant to be consumed.*

## How to use the oils

When added to a bath, the oils are used neat, pouring the required amount in the running water, which disperses and mixes them. If they are being used for massage they should be mixed into a neutral carrier oil.

Essential oils should be stored, individually or in combinations, in clean glass containers – dark glass if possible, sealed tightly and kept away from light and heat.

The various properties of each oil and combinations of oils given below can help you select the one(s) most useful for your present state of health.

BASIL an antiseptic as well as an antidepressant and a tonic for the digestion. On its own it can be used (20 drops in a bath) to treat weakness, fatigue (including mental tiredness/ fogginess), headaches, nausea, feelings of tension or faintness and depression.

CHAMOMILE a soothing agent, sleep-enhancer, digestive and general tonic, pain-reliever and an antibacterial agent. It can be used on its own (20 drops in a bath) to treat sleep and digestive disturbances, skin conditions, neuralgia and inflammation. It soothes tired and irritated eyes when used as a compress or eyewash. Combined with sage it can be used to ease menopausal problems (add 10 drops of each to your bath).

CYPRESS an astringent, antispasmodic tonic and also useful as a deodorant. It can be used alone (20 drops in a bath) to treat rheumatic and muscular conditions, coughs, flu and nervous tension. Combined with lavender (add 20 drops of each to a warm bath) it is useful for menopausal problems or as a general treatment for the nervous system.

LAVENDER an antispasmodic, antiseptic and general 'restorative'. Use it alone (20 drops in a bath) when you are stressed or to treat nervous problems or headache. Use it with cypress (as above) for menopausal or 'nervous system' problems, and with vetiver for anxiety (10 drops of each).

NEROLI an antidepressant, antiseptic, digestive aid as well as being said to be both a sedative and aphrodisiac. Use it alone (20 drops in a bath) to treat depression, insomnia and nervous tension, digestive upsets and lack of sexual interest. Try it together with basil (10 drops of each in a bath) in cases of anxiety, tension or depression.

## SUPPLEMENTATION TO HELP SLEEP AND THE PRODUCTION OF THE GROWTH HORMONE

### Tryptophan
The amino acid tryptophan is no longer available over the counter as a supplement, after a contaminated batch from Japan caused severe toxic reactions. A safe form of tryptophan can be obtained at health food stores as 5-hydroxy-l-tryptophan (5-HTP) – this is discussed below.

The plant proteins in chlorella and other blue-green algae (available in most healthfood stores) are ideal sources of tryptophan; a drink containing these in the evening will provide enough to aid sleep, as would a few grams of full-spectrum amino acid powder (capsules or powder, also available in healthfood stores).

### Melatonin
Plant sources of this hormone help to induce sleep and relieve depression. 2-3 mg taken before bedtime are suggested.

### Calcium and Magnesium
These, in a ratio of 2:1, are also useful relaxing nutrients. A gram of calcium and half a gram of magnesium (tablet, capsule, powder or liquid) taken at night helps the relaxation process.

**Arginine and Ornithine**

CAUTIONS

*If either arginine or ornithine is taken, it should be for a period of two to three months only, with a similar rest period before starting again. This is suggested to prevent imbalances developing in the amino acid content in the body. These growth hormone stimulators should never be taken (unless under supervision) by anyone who has not yet completed their growth phase. The skin may become coarse if excessive growth hormone is released.*

These amino acids are used by devotees of life-extension programmes to produce growth hormone release. On balance, ornithine is preferred by experts in this area of nutrition, with 2 grams taken in the morning and 2 grams taken in the evening, not at meal times, being the standard recommendation. When arginine is taken, the recommended dose is twice that for ornithine.

A supplement of antioxidants (vitamins A, C and E with selenium) is suggested as a useful accompaniment to these amino acids.

**5-HTP (5-hydroxy-l-tryptophan) for serotonin and sleep enhancement**

Tryptophan is an amino acid which has been used to treat stress symptoms and insomnia for many years. It was removed from the market in the early 1990s, as mentioned above, when Japanese manufacturers used a genetically-engineered bacterial process to produce tryptophan, leading to major health problems.

A plant source of a form of tryptophan (5-HTP) is found in a bean (*Griffonia simplicifolia*) which grows in Africa. Research has confirmed that 5-HTP is at least as effective as tryptophan (and probably more so) and that it converts into serotonin when it reaches the brain. Serotonin deficit is thought by many experts to be a major feature of fibromyalgia – see 'Brain Changes' in Chapter 2, page 32 (I. Caruso *et al.*, 1990).

## Chemical Sensitivities

These are often associated with candidiasis (yeast) infections (see more below) and with chronic stress and toxicity problems. The factors that help restore normal function – a sound diet, exercise, rest and relaxation, detoxification and so on – will all help to reduce the tendency towards chemical sensitivity. Supplementation with antioxidant nutrients such as vitamins C (1 to 3 grams daily), E (400 iu daily), selenium (200 mcg daily) and zinc (15 to 30 mg daily) can be useful in helping to increase the body's tolerance of chemicals, as well as neutralizing many of their harmful oxidation effects.

## Candidiasis

Complete the Candida Questionnaire in Chapter 2 (page 35). If this indicates a likelihood of yeast-overgrowth, you are strongly urged to seek advice from a suitably qualified health care professional. Specific tests may be needed to confirm the condition.

The anti-Candida measures outlined below may prove useful in the case of an established yeast-overgrowth, and should be continued for no fewer than three months, and possibly longer depending on the response.

### AN ANTI-CANDIDA STRATEGY

- With each meal (three times a day), take one strong caprylic acid capsule (this is an antifungal coconut plant extract) and one high-potency garlic supplement.
- To encourage a repopulation of intestinal flora, between meals (three times daily) take *acidophilus* and *bifidobacteria* (powder or capsule form). General nutritional support is also useful, so take a soundly formulated, yeast-free multivitamin/multimineral supplement to provide at least the recommended daily allowances of the major nutrients (Chaitow and Trenev, 1990, Chaitow, 1991).

- Chew well, eat slowly and try not to drink much with meals. Eat three small main meals daily and two snack meals, where possible (but do not make the snacks sugar-rich foods), or take 3 to 5 grams of a full-spectrum amino acid complex between main meals, twice daily (see under 'Fatigue', below).
- Avoid, as far as possible, *all* refined sugars and, for the first few weeks, avoid very sweet fruits as well (such as melons and sweet grapes). Also avoid aged cheeses, dried fruits and any food obviously derived from or containing yeast.
- Avoid caffeine-containing drinks and foods (coffee, tea, chocolate, cola) as these produce a sugar release that is not desirable where yeast has proliferated. Avoid alcohol, too. This suggestion is something to try to do, but it may be difficult when you are with other people, so do not be obsessive about it, just careful.

Expect to feel off-colour for the first week of such a programme as the yeast 'die-off' takes place.

Note that other antifungal substances are available and may be more effective in certain cases than following the suggestions above. However, the strategy is usually beneficial if it is maintained for several months. My book *Candida Albicans – Could Yeast Be Your Problem?* (Thorsons) is recommended for more details of appropriate anti-yeast strategies.

## Depression

The stress-reduction and detoxification methods described above and below, as well as the strategies given to treat candidiasis and viral problems, if you suffer these, can improve your health to such a level that your reactive depression symptoms reduce. As life becomes more meaningful and a sense of control is restored, so depression tends to fade away.

If depression is a *primary* factor, then this may need to be dealt with using appropriate medication. Certainly, the evidence is overwhelming that low doses of tricyclic antidepressant medication helps many fibromyalgia patients, probably because sleep patterns are improved. The hydrotherapy, autogenic and other methods described in this chapter are also all likely to be helpful in this respect.

### Fatigue

Fatigue can be the result of a number of problems, and the strategies required to tackle it will vary depending on its cause. Here are some of the most common causes, and ways in which you can deal with them.

### ALLERGIES

The stress-reduction, allergy-coping and detoxification methods described in this chapter are three of the key ways in which allergies can be overcome and, as a result, there will be an enhancement of energy.

In one study of what was called 'the allergic tension-fatigue syndrome', it was found that, of 50 people suffering from tension and fatigue, 75 per cent of them had a history of nasal, ocular, respiratory or skin allergies. Over half of them received treatment in the form of elimination diets (see under 'Allergies' above for more on what these are), with excellent results.

### DEFICIENCIES

Professor Melvyn Werbach of UCLA has shown that nutritional deficiencies of potassium, magnesium, iron, folic acid, pantothenic acid (vitamin $B_5$), pyridoxine ($B_6$), $B_{12}$, vitamin C, zinc, aspartic acid, the amino acids carnitine, glutamine, inosine and co-enzyme Q10 induce chronic fatigue (1990).

Taking supplements of vitamins and minerals for which there is a deficiency can help restore energy levels.

## LOW BLOOD SUGAR

The brain depends on two key 'nutrients': blood sugar and oxygen. The discussion on hyperventilation has already shown how inadequate circulation to the brain can starve it of oxygen.

If there is also a tendency to low blood sugar, this can make hyperventilation symptoms far worse, making fatigue and 'brain fog' infinitely more marked.

The solution to low blood sugar problems is NOT to increase sugar intake!

Safe and helpful strategies are described below, but first it is necessary to see whether low blood sugar is part of your problem.

### Low blood sugar questionnaire ?

Answers to the following questions will indicate whether this is a likely feature of your condition.

1  On waking in the morning do you feel lethargic?

2  Before mealtime do you frequently feel
   shaky, lightheaded, faint, irritable?

3  Do you get a lift in energy after a meal?

4  Do you crave sugar-rich foods, or carbohydrate-
   laden foods (cakes, cookies, pasta, bread)?

5  Does your energy 'crash' late morning or late afternoon?

6  Do you regularly 'use' tea, coffee, cola drinks, chocolate,
   (and/or tobacco products) to gain a lift from 'energy blues'?

7  If you were to miss a meal, or if it was delayed for an hour
   or more, would you feel unwell?

If you've answered YES to two or more of these questions, you may well suffer from a low blood sugar tendency, and if there is such a tendency it may well be characterized by mood swings, sugar and stimulant craving, a feeling of being spaced out and anxious if meals are missed, as well as fatigue. It is usually possible to rebalance this tendency, but as an initial strategy it may be helpful to introduce, twice daily, between meals, 4 to 5 grams of full-spectrum amino acid complex, in powder or capsule form, in order to help stabilize blood sugar fluctuations and decrease sugar-craving episodes (Davies, 1987).

To help achieve a more balanced management of blood sugar, it is also suggested that a supplement be taken that contains what is known as Glucose Tolerance Factor, incorporating the vital nutrient chromium (200 mcg daily).

Eating six small meals a day is more advisable than sticking to three meals or fewer a day.

It is very important to avoid sugar and stimulants (caffeine and alcohol in particular) and to concentrate on eating adequate protein.

Also, the constitutional hydrotherapy methods described in Chapter 7 and the restoration of normal breathing (see the exercise under Anti-arousal Breathing Technique, page 135) should be central elements in the treatment of all fatigue sufferers.

### Inflammation and pain

While it is clear that so-called fibrositis does not involve active inflammation, many of the associated muscle, soft-tissue and joint problems involving pain certainly do. The dietary strategies outlined below are effective and safe and can be incorporated into a normal eating pattern without difficulty.

There are two major anti-inflammatory nutritional methods that are useful in most pain situations:

1 the dietary approach
2 the enzyme approach
   — both or either can be used if appropriate.

## WHEN ARE THESE METHODS APPROPRIATE?

Inflammation is a natural and mostly useful bodily response to irritation, injury and infection. It can be a major part of the process of getting better, despite the fact that it is not exactly pleasant. So, to drastically alter or reduce inflammation may be counterproductive and actually a mistake, as has been shown to be the case when arthritis has been treated by means of non-steroidal anti-inflammatory drugs over 30 years or so – untreated joints have been shown to be healthier than those that have been treated.

If you want to use nutritional tactics for reducing inflammation, this option should first be discussed with a healthcare professional and it should be agreed that this is a safe way forward.

If pain is reduced where inflammation exists, it is a mistake to then become very active, if this involves stressing a previously inflamed or damaged area. Remember that overuse of damaged areas (joint surfaces) is one of the reasons for arthritic joints worsening when the pain is eased by drugs.

So, it is suggested that safe anti-inflammatory methods (see below) are used with common sense. Never overdo any activity just because the pain eases, if the area is still healing or inflamed.

It is always safer to seek professional advice rather than just hope for the best in such matters.

## DIETARY APPROACHES

### Reduce consumption of animal fats

Inflammation and pain processes involve minute chemical substances your body makes, called prostaglandins and leukotrienes. These, in turn, are to a great extent dependent on the presence of arachidonic acid, which the body manufactures mainly from animal fats. This means that reducing your intake of animal fats cuts down your access to the enzymes that help to produce arachidonic acid, thereby reducing the levels of the inflammatory substances released in tissues which contribute so greatly to pain. Achieving this end, then, is the first priority in an anti-inflammatory dietary approach, which means cutting down or eliminating as much as possible the amount of fat in your diet. To do this, adopt the following guidelines:

- eat fat-free or low-fat milk, yogurt and cheese rather than full-fat varieties, and avoid butter altogether
- avoid meat fat completely and, since much of the fat in meat is invisible, meat itself can be left out of the diet for a time (or permanently); the skin of poultry should be avoided
- look for fats mentioned in the ingredients given on the packaging of products such as biscuits and other manufactured foods, and avoid those containing fats.

## Consume more fish oils

Some fish – mainly those that come from cold water areas such as the North Sea – contain high levels of eicosapentenoic acid (EPA). This reduces the levels of arachidonic acid in the tissues of the body and, therefore, helps to ensure that there is a reduction in the inflammatory substances produced. Further, and very importantly, fish oil has these anti-inflammatory effects without interfering with the useful jobs that some prostaglandins do, such as protecting the delicate lining of the stomach and maintaining the correct level of blood clotting. This last feature is a key one, because there are many drugs that can do just what fish oil can do (reducing inflammation and therefore pain), but, unfortunately they can do so only by also causing new problems. EPA does not do this, unless you happen to be allergic to fish.

Research has shown that when EPA is taken for rheumatic and arthritic conditions, it offers relief from swelling, stiffness and pain, although these benefits do not usually become evident until three months after fish oil supplements have begun to be taken, reaching their most effective level after around six months (Werbach, 1991).

If you want to follow this strategy:

- eat fish such as herring, sardines, salmon and mackerel at least twice weekly – and more often if you wish
- take 10 to 15 EPA capsules a day at regular intervals when the inflammation is at its worst, and continue to do so until relief appears. Then take a maintenance dose of six daily.

## Boost pain relief with DL-phenylalanine (DLPA)

Amino acids are parts of protein that are natural elements of the body's environment, used to manufacture new tissues and cells.

When taken individually as supplements, amino acids can have special effects, as is the case with DL-phenylalanine (DLPA), which has been shown to have painkilling potential under certain circumstances. For example, when a person is having some other form of treatment, such as taking painkillers (say, aspirin) or having acupuncture, taking DLPA at the same time can make the treatment more effective. If it is taken on its own, it does not seem to have much effect, but when it is combined with another approach it makes the treatment more successful.

Doses recommended for helping potentiate pain relief in this way are in the region of 2 to 3 grams daily, in divided doses, not taken at mealtimes.

## Use enzymes as anti-inflammatories

Enzymes are minute chemical substances that take part in or commence all the chemical reactions that take place in the body, and so they are vital for life itself. Some of these are very involved in the process of digestion, such as protease.

It has been found that taking other protein-digesting enzymes derived from plants as supplements has a gentle but substantial anti-inflammatory influence. Such supplements include bromelaine, which comes from the pineapple plant, and papain, from the papaya plant. It is necessary to ensure that around 2 to 3 grams of one or the other (bromelaine is the more effective of the two) are taken each day at regular points other than mealtimes (or else all it will do is help digest your food) as part of an anti-inflammatory, pain-relieving strategy.

### Don't drink instant coffee

It has been found that coffee contains substances that block the receptor sites used by our natural painkilling endorphins, making pain seem more intense. This has only been found to be true for instant rather than brewed forms of coffee. This is not a recommendation to drink filter and other coffee, but rather a suggestion that at least instant coffee should be avoided by people in pain.

### Irritable bowel syndrome (IBS)

Allergic symptoms need to be considered and dealt with (as we saw under 'Allergies', above).

The most common sensitivities are to grains (wheat especially), corn, yeasts, food colourings, coffee, citrus and dairy products. 'Safe' foods are usually lamb, fresh white fish, cabbage, peas, carrots, rye-based biscuits or crispbreads (not those made from wheat), rice cakes, milk-free margarine and weak black tea.

Candidiasis (discussed above) is a common cause of irritable bowel, as are parasites (the commonest is *Giardia lamblia*), which need to be dealt with by expertly applied medication.

Hydrochloric acid deficiencies are common in sufferers of Irritable Bowel Syndrome, as are deficiencies of digestive enzymes. Expert advice is required to help normalize such problems, but taking supplements of pro-biotic substances such as *acidophilus*, *bifidobacteria* and *L. bulgaricus* – all in dairy-free preparations if possible – is a safe and effective way of starting to return the bowels to normal healthy functioning (Chaitow and Trenev, 1990, Chaitow, 1991).

Enteric-coated peppermint oil capsules, and Aloe vera extracts, can both help to sooth the cramps so common in IBS.

The detoxification programme outlined (see page 162), plus the stress-reduction methods mentioned earlier in this chapter, are all recommended as adjuncts to any other forms of treatment.

## Memory and concentration ('brain-fog')

The autogenic training exercise on page 138, combined with the anti-arousal breathing techniques described on page 135, are two excellent ways in which you can start to improve the circulation to and through the brain. Better blood sugar balance is also vital. In addition, the constitutional hydrotherapy method described in Chapter 7 and the bodywork approaches and stretching exercises described in Chapter 8 will further improve this.

Dealing with any thyroid imbalance, allergies, toxicity, candidiasis or viral problems that also exist is a further boost to normalizing brain function, as all of these can cause or aggravate the typical symptoms.

A herbal approach, involving the taking of standardized extracts of the plant *Ginkgo biloba*, is suggested for a six-month trial period. This has been shown in medical studies (where doses of between 120 and 240 mg were taken daily) to improve memory and reduce the symptoms of inadequate circulation to the brain (Foster, 1991, Kleijnen, 1992, Schaffer, 1985, Vorberg, 1985).

This herb has no side-effects and can be taken by anyone. It is now one of the most prescribed medications in Germany and Scandinavia for cerebral dysfunction – specifically for dizziness, memory loss, tinnitus, headaches and emotional instability combined with anxiety. It is also used for treating inadequate peripheral circulation (where someone has cold hands and feet).

In addition, to further boost the circulation, not less than 90 mg of the nutrient co-enzyme Q10 can be taken. This takes up to a month before being effective in enhancing oxygen transportation. This supplement is also useful in the treatment of fatigue, according to numerous (mainly Japanese and Dutch) trials (Kamikawa, 1985, Elsevier, 1980, Vanfraechem, 1981).

I have personal experience of their benefits, as I have been prescribing both these substances for people with chronic fatigue syndrome (ME) and fibromyalgia for several years, with excellent results. Remember that it is slow acting and improvement before three months is unlikely.

## Pain

See under 'Anxiety' and 'Inflammation and Pain' above, and also Chapters 8 and 9.

## Premenstrual tension syndrome (PMT or PMS)

Dr. G. Abraham has treated premenstrual symptoms and classifies them into the following categories (Werbach, 1991).

### 'A' for anxiety

The symptoms being nervous tension, mood swings, irritability, anxiety and insomnia. They stem from elevated levels of oestrogen and low levels of progesterone and, usually, a tendency towards a diet high in sugar and dairy foods. The nutritional treatment for this group of symptoms is to take between 200 and 800 mg of vitamin $B_6$ daily (the high dosage should be taken under expert guidance only) to reduce blood oestrogen levels and increase progesterone. It is useful to take omega-6 fatty acids (either as borage oil, flaxseed oil or evening primrose oil) in doses of 1 to 2 grams daily. All caffeine and sugar intake should be reduced or eliminated for at least three days prior to the onset of premenstrual symptoms, and dairy products (and calcium) cut back.

## 'C' for craving

The symptoms are headaches, cravings for sweets, increased appetite, pounding heart, dizziness or fainting, fatigue. This form of PMT is associated with poor carbohydrate tolerance, low blood magnesium levels and possible prostaglandin imbalances. The nutritional treatment for this group of symptoms is to take magnesium supplements – at least 500 mg daily (usually a combination of 1 gram of calcium and ½ gram of magnesium is suggested). Also useful is the taking of omega-6 fatty acids (either as borage oil, flaxseed oil or evening primrose oil) in doses of 1 to 2 grams daily. Also, all caffeine and sugar intake must be reduced or eliminated and the amount of salt consumed should be reduced to not more than 3 grams a day for at least three days prior to the onset of premenstrual symptoms.

## 'D' for depression

The symptoms here are depression, forgetfulness, tearfulness and confusion. This form of PMT stems from high levels of progesterone during the mid-cycle ovulation phase, and sometimes elevated adrenal androgens (in hairy people). Sometimes lead toxicity seems to be involved in this type of PMT. Expert advice is required once the individual hormonal pattern has been established, but caffeine should be reduced or eliminated and taking vitamin E (300 to 600 iu daily for at least two months initially, to assess its effect), plus omega-6 fatty acids (either as borage oil, flaxseed oil or evening primrose oil) in doses of 1 to 2 grams daily should help.

## 'H' for hyperhydration

The symptoms are weight gain of more than 1.3 kg/3 lb, swelling of the extremities, breast tenderness and abdominal bloating. These symptoms are the result of fluid retention, which may be due to elevated levels of aldosterone. This substance can be reduced by taking vitamin $B_6$ supplements (500 mg daily, under the supervision of a healthcare professional). Another option, also to be followed under medical supervision only, is to take between 200,000 and 300,000 iu daily of vitamin A, which has been shown to help this form of PMT if taken from day 15 of the menstrual cycle until the onset of the symptoms. Do note, however, that vitamin A can be toxic in high doses and must not be taken during pregnancy. Also found to be useful in clinical trials has been omega-6 fatty acids (either as borage oil, flaxseed oil or evening primrose oil) in doses of 1 to 2 grams daily. Vitamin E can usually help reduce breast symptoms (300 to 600 iu daily), though in some studies the symptoms actually worsened. Also, salt intake must be kept low – 3 grams daily at most.

### Thyroid support

In Chapter 2, details were provided of thyroid hormone imbalances and the suggested FMS connection.

The questionnaire (page 55) and the 'underarm temperature test' described in that chapter provide clues as to possible thyroid involvement in your condition.

There are several general strategies which can enhance thyroid function even in the absence of actual thyroid hormone replacement, which requires specialist medical knowledge and experience.

Dr. Joseph Pizzorno, founder president of Bastyr University (Seattle) and author of the excellent book *Total Wellness* (Prima), recommends iodine, stating, 'Low thyroid activity is a common problem and much can be done to help reestablish adequate thyroid function. The first step . . . is to ensure that the body is producing enough thyroid hormone. This requires an adequate intake of iodine because the mineral is used to form the thyroid hormones.'

- Supplementation with products such as Thorne Research's *Iodine and Tyrosine* capsules (2 daily) is a useful way of achieving an adequate intake.

- Good iodine-rich foods include sea vegetables such as kelp, dulse, nori, wakame, kombu (available from specialist delicatessen stores, Japanese food stores, some health food stores) and saltwater fish, as well as iodized salt.

Some health-enhancing foods can actually have a negative effect on the thyroid. These are known as *goitrogens* and include: all vegetables from the brassica family when raw – cabbage, turnips, cauliflower, broccoli and radishes – as well as cassava, soybeans, pine nuts, millet and peanuts. The goitrogenic effect of these vegetables is reduced if they are cooked.

Vitamins A, B-complex and C as well as the mineral zinc are helpful in supporting thyroid function. Supplementation should ideally be under guidance from a qualified nutritional expert. Zinc is commonly deficient in the modern diet and it is an essential substance for the formation of enzymes which convert thyroid hormone into its active form. An adequate dosage of zinc is 20 mg daily.

Selenium is also an essential nutrient which when deficient seems to encourage thyroid dysfunction. An adequate dosage of selenium is 150 mcg.

Iron and copper deficiencies may also play a part in thyroid imbalance. Supplementation of these should be based on advice from a qualified nutritional expert.

Exercise is extremely helpful in enhancement of thyroid function. Aerobic exercise encourages thyroid hormone secretion and is recommended three times weekly for not less than 20 minutes.

## Toxicity

Toxicity can be usefully reduced by following a pattern of regular detoxification days, as outlined below.

Among the most important detoxification functions of the body are performed by the liver, and support for this organ may be needed to ensure adequate detoxification functions.

Other techniques you can use to help you in this task are hydrotherapy methods, skin brushing, sauna baths, aerobic exercise, specific herbal liver treatments and bodywork, to assist in lymphatic drainage.

Some safe self-help measures are described below, but if toxicity is a factor in your condition, advice from an appropriately qualified health care professional should be sought.

It is known from research that *everyone* has deposits of DDT, lead, cadmium and dioxins in their bodies – none of which should be in any of us. The chances are, therefore, that a wide range of petrochemical by-products, as well as heavy metals, food additives, colourings, flavourings, preservatives, insecticides and pesticides are also present in most of us.

We have become filters and traps for pollutants that exist in ever greater amounts all around us, and these have a definite effect on our overall health, as well as imposing ever greater demands on the organs that are responsible for eliminating harmful substances from the body.

The toxic build-up in our bodies is greater when we are stressed. Take one simple example. If muscles are held tensely, they create and retain acid wastes. These can be flushed away by exercise and fresh oxygenated blood, and they can also be excreted through the skin as sweat. If they are not eliminated from the body in these ways, they are retained in the tissues due to sluggish circulation, poor oxygenation caused by inadequate exercise, and inadequate breathing.

All the organs of detoxification need to be well nourished in order to work efficiently. They need to be well supplied with fresh oxygenated blood carrying adequate nutrient supplies and served by a nervous system that is working correctly.

As we get older, the body's cleansing systems, those that detoxify the body, become less efficient, as do the various supporting functions such as circulation and elimination. Whatever age we are, though, we all carry greater or lesser loads of undesirable debris in our tissues. These amounts are added to daily by exposure to new toxic materials in food, water and the air we breathe, not to forget any extra toxicity we create or acquire through infection or from certain forms of medication.

No one has a clear idea of just what damage all this is doing to us. The problem is complicated by the fact that there are very real individual biochemical differences we are each born with, and huge differences exist between people's levels of nutritional, structural and emotional excellence or deficiency. However, we know that although some people handle the toxic load better than others, all of us are negatively affected – sometimes with profound consequences.

The best way of handling this sort of situation is to decrease the toxic burden, to encourage the body to eliminate more and to find ways of reducing future build-ups of toxic substances.

## HELPING YOURSELF DETOXIFY

Not only can we ensure that we eat a balanced diet, we can make sure we get enough of the right sorts of exercise. Also, we can try to boost that vital area of our mental well-being which has such an influence on everything else – our emotional and stress-coping functions. Fortunately, a number of safe methods exist that can encourage the body to eliminate impurities. These include repetitive, short fasting periods, which allow the liver in particular to recover from toxic stress. Of special relevance to fibromyalgia is the fact that on short fasts, growth hormone production is stimulated (Kernt, 1982, Weindruch and Walford, 1988, Chaitow, 1992, Kenton, 1988).

# GENTLE DETOXIFICATION AND DIETARY PROGRAMMES

## CAUTION

*If you are a recovering drug user or alcoholic or have an eating disorder, are markedly frail or underweight, have diabetes or are pregnant, then you should not use the following programme without consulting a health care professional about it first. If you have Candida overgrowth or bowel problems, then self-help and/or professional guidance on normalizing your situation should be followed before using the detoxification methods below.*

If someone is robust and vital, they will need a more vigorous detoxi fication programme than will someone who is unwell and somewhat fragile in health. The following detoxification programme is safe for almost everyone.

### Liver support

Before and during detoxification it is important to offer support to the liver. This marvellous and complicated organ conducts over 500 different detoxification processes which basically prevent each of us from drowning in our own toxins. To help the liver, some very simple strategies are recommended.

- Ensure a high intake of garlic and onions.
- Take a supplement of the herb *Silybum marianum* (milk thistle): 120 mg three times a day.
- If possible, include artichoke and dandelion greens in the diet as these two plants are very supportive of liver function. Alternatively, seek out a herbal combination which includes these (artichoke, dandelion) as well as Turmeric and catechin extracts.
- Include in the diet a high intake of brassica family (cabbage, etc.) – but not raw if thyroid is a problem (see notes on Thyroid Support in this chapter, page 159).

- Supplement with the amino acid compound reduced glutathione (100 mg daily away from mealtimes).
- Undertake periodic short-term fasting – as described later in this chapter.
- Use a sauna to enhance elimination once or twice weekly (unless this is too exhausting).

## Detoxification by dietary means

Over almost every weekend for a few months (and thereafter once a month at least), choose between the following options.

- *A short, water-only fast* This lasts 24 to 36 hours and is to be conducted over a weekend (starting Friday evening and ending Saturday evening or Sunday morning, or just all day Saturday, so that work schedules are not interfered with). Make sure that not less than 2 litres (4 pints) and not more than 4.5 litres (8 pints) of water are consumed during the day. After fasting for 24 to 36 hours, break the fast with stewed pears or apples (with no added sweetening) or a light vegetable soup, or plain, low-fat, unsweetened yogurt. On the Sunday have a raw food day, eating fruit and salads only, chewing the food well, plus glasses of water. Alternatively, if you have a sensitive digestion, eat lightly cooked (steamed or stir-fried) vegetables, baked potatoes and stewed fruit (with no added sugar) plus yogurt.
- *A full weekend monodiet* Start on Friday night and go through to Sunday evening eating only a single food. Have up to 1.3 kg/3 lb daily of any single fruit you like, such as grapes, apples, pears (the latter being the best choice if you have a history of allergies) or papaya (this is ideal if you have digestive problems). You can eat it all raw or lightly stewed, without sweetening it. Alternatively, have up to 0.5 kg/1 lb (dry weight) of brown rice, buckwheat or millet daily, or up to 1.3 kg/3

lb of potatoes (skin and all) daily, boiled and eaten whenever desired. The grains can be made palatable by adding a little lemon juice and olive oil.

Whichever option you choose, make sure you rest and keep warm and have no plans for any activities of any kind, as this is a time to allow all available energy to focus on the repairing and cleansing processes of detoxification.

In between these weekend detoxification intensives, you can institute a milder midweek programme of detoxification in the following way.

- *For breakfast* Fresh fruit (raw or lightly cooked with no sweetening) and live yogurt, or home-made muesli (seeds and nuts and grains) and live yogurt, or cooked grains (buckwheat, millet, linseed, barley, rice and so on) and yogurt. To drink, choose from herbal tea (linden blossom, chamomile, mint, sage or lemon verbena) or simply have lemon and hot water.
- *For a light lunch or supper* One of these should be a raw salad with jacket potato or brown rice, and either bean curd (tofu) or low-fat cheese or nuts/seeds. Alternatively, if raw foods cause digestive problems, have a stir-fried vegetable/tofu meal or steamed vegetables with potatoes or rice together with low-fat cheese or nuts/seeds.
- *For your main meal* Choose between fish, chicken, game or vegetarian savoury mixtures (pulse/grain combinations) and accompany this with vegetables that have been lightly steamed, baked or stir-fried.
- *Desserts* Lightly stewed fruit, sweetened with a little apple or lemon juice, not sugar, or live natural yogurt.
- *Seasonings* Use garlic and herbs, avoiding salt as much as possible.

Eat slowly, chew well, don't drink with meals and consume at least 1 litre (2 pints) of liquid daily between meals.

Other forms of detoxification are being researched. For example, noted nutritional expert Dr. Jeffrey Bland has formulated a meal-replacement product (Ultra-Clear) which is based on rice protein, and which is also rich in detoxifying nutrients. By combining avoidance of allergenic foods and using products such as this, a modified fast/detoxification programme can be carried out while continuing with normal activities. Research has shown this to be very helpful for many people with FMS/CFS.

A study of Bland's detoxification methods involved 106 patients at different clinics, with either CFS or FMS (plus IBS). The programme called for avoidance of known food allergens, encouragement of intestinal repair, stimulation of liver detoxification and a modified fast using the rice protein powder. Over a 10-week period there was a greater than 50 per cent reduction in symptoms as well as laboratory evidence of improved liver and digestive function (J. Bland, 1995).

Joseph Pizzorno ND, one of America's leading naturopathic physicians and Founder President of Bastyr University, Seattle, encourages liver detoxification in such cases by means of increased eating of brassica family foods (cabbage, etc.), the use of specific nutrients such as N-acetyl-cysteine and glutathione, as well as taking the herb *Silybum marianum* (milk thistle) – 120 mg three times daily. He also encourages adrenal gland function (supplementing with vitamins C and $B_5$). He states, 'The strong correlation between chronic fatigue syndrome, fibromyalgia and multiple chemical sensitivities suggests that all may respond to hepatic [liver] detoxification, food allergy control and a gut restoration diet' (J. Pizzorno, 1996).

## What to expect during detoxification

In the early days (for the first few weekends of short-term fasting or a monodiet) you could develop a headache and furred tongue.

These are side-effects of the detoxification process and tell you that it is working. They slowly become less noticeable as detoxification progresses weekend by weekend.

It is important that you take nothing to stop the headache, but just rest as much as you can.

As the weeks pass, your skin should become clearer (it may be a bit spotty for a while at the start, but this is another little sign that the detoxification is working), your eyes clearer, brain sharper, digestion more efficient and your energy levels should start to rise.

When the tongue no longer becomes furred and headaches no longer appear, the fasts or monodiets can be spread further apart – to three a month and then two a month and then a maintenance detoxification once a month.

When a definite change is noticed and there is far less reaction to the weekend fasts, the in-between, milder detoxification pattern can also be relaxed a bit, and a few 'naughty but nice' tasty toxins can be taken from time to time. By this time your own internal detoxification system should be able to cope with such indiscretions!

## ENHANCING DETOXIFICATION

### Skin brushing-the dry methods

This is best done 'dry', before you wash, shower or bathe, and it need take only a few minutes (five at most). Once you decide to start using skin brushing to improve your skin and health, you should also make up your mind that it will become a daily routine for maximum effect.

### PREPARATION

Choose a warm, draught-free room, and undress. Have a stool ready, as sitting makes it easier to get to hard-to-reach areas like the backs of the legs without having to get into all sorts of contortions. You will also need a bath-mit, loofah or a natural bristle body-brush.

## METHOD

- Start brushing the skin gently, and expect at first what is called a 'red reaction', which shows that your circulation is responding to the stimulation you are giving it. The action of brushing needs to be circular, 'creeping' and firm but not irritating. The circular motion helps you avoid rubbing over one area too much (at first once or twice over any part of the skin is adequate) and the 'creeping' movement has the same effect. By this term is meant that you simply gradually move from where you are presently circling to the next area, not by lifting the brush but by altering the direction as you make the circular motion, sliding gently towards the next part of the skin due to be brushed.
- Pay particular attention to the skin on the backs of the legs and arms, as well as your back, abdomen and chest, where you may be more sensitive and tender. Women should avoid brushing the breast tissue and be very gentle on the inner thighs. Again, it is important that you start slowly and gently!

After a week or so of daily skin brushing, the skin that was tender will be less so and you can slowly increase the pressure and vigour of your brushing.

If there are bits of your back you cannot reach, use a dry towel to briskly rub these – it will not be as effective as a brush, mit or loofah, but will be better than no friction at all.

### Skinbrushing – the wet method

Choose a mit, loofah or natural bristle skin brush as before, but this time have a shower or bath and, before drying yourself, brush the skin as above but moisten the mit, loofah or brush. Shower afterwards to get rid of surface skin that has been loosened by the process, ideally finishing with water that is around body temperature or slightly cooler.

### The salt glow

'This essentially involves rubbing wet sea salt or Epsom salts over the body. It is particularly beneficial for people who have difficulty sweating or who have poor circulation to their hands and/or feet, and for people prone to rheumatic aches and pains, so it is ideal for people with fibromyalgia.

It is best if someone else rubs the salt over you – if you try to do this yourself, you have to accept that you will be unable to reach parts of your body. Unlike the skin-brushing method, which should become part of your daily routine, the salt glow is something to look forward to now and again – perhaps once a week at most if you have difficulty sweating; once a month or so for general detoxification purposes.

PREPARATION

To give yourself a salt glow rub, you will need a bowl and at least 225 g (8 oz) of coarse salt or Epsom salt.

METHOD

- Sit on a stool in the bath or shower and add water to the salt in the bowl to moisten it – just enough to make the salt crystals stick together.
- Take a small amount of wet salt in each hand (about a tablespoonful) and, starting with one foot, work the salt over the skin, rubbing up and down the leg using circular motions. Try to rub firmly, even vigorously, skin that is usually exposed, such as the legs, as you apply the damp

salt; ensure that all the skin gets some rubbing and some salt. Work up each leg and then do each arm.

- Next, work salt onto/into the skin around your back without straining yourself (if a partner is handy, they could usefully do all the rubbing here for you). Then, apply the salt (rubbing firmly but not irritatingly) to the abdomen and chest and up to the neck (women should avoid the breast tissue).

- After the salt rub, shower thoroughly, ideally using a hand shower and warm water to cleanse the surface of the skin. As you are doing this and the water is playing on a given area, use your free hand to rub the salt and water off the skin, giving the area a bit more of a rub as you do so. Dry yourself with a vigorous towelling down and go to bed (make sure the bed and the room are warm).

You should sleep well, and may perspire heavily the first few times you have a salt glow. Have water by the bed in case you get thirsty. As your skin becomes more efficient, any heavy perspiration will lessen as time passes.

This is a wonderful skin tonic and detoxification method.

## Viral infection

Herbal anti-viral medicines, such as echinacea, hydrastis and berberine, plus a host of other anti-viral products from Chinese and Western traditions, can be safely used as powerful anti-viral agents, ideally taken under expert supervision. The general detoxification and immune-enhancing methods discussed above should also enable the body to handle viral challenges adequately once more.

Specific strategies exist in which nutritional patterns which inhibit certain viruses (notably the herpes group) can be used, by tilting the diet towards a lysine-rich pattern and away from arginine-rich foods, while also supplementing it with the amino acid lysine. Such strategies, though, need to be formulated and prescribed individually (Balch, 1990, Chaitow [ed.], 1994).

### Scars and trigger point pain
A number of researchers have shown that careful evaluation of tissues around scars, even old ones, can reveal active trigger points that may be deactivated manually, or by needling (acupuncture). The 'quality' of pain from such scars is often sharp/cutting/burning rather than the deep ache of trigger points elsewhere in the body (Kobesova *et al.*, 2007).

# 7

# Constitutional (Non-specific) Treatment Methods

When we treat a symptom or a condition by specific means – say taking a painkilling substance for a pain, or an anti-inflammatory agent for an inflammation or an indigestion tablet for indigestion – there is a clear expectation that you will feel better, that the symptoms will be modified, changed, masked or removed. There is no sense in any of these actions that the cause of the pain, the inflammation or the stomach ache, is being dealt with, only that the *effects* are being taken care of, possibly for the short term and probably with side-effects, albeit mild ones.

This is a choice that is constantly being made in medicine, and the balance between benefit and side-effect is always the trade-off . As long as these negatives are not of great consequence, we can usually live with this in return for the short-term gain of less pain or discomfort. We might have a debate about whether or not there are more efficient and/or less undesirable ways of treating unpleasant symptoms, but, in the main, whether you use an over-the-counter medication, a herbal medicine, a nutritional supplement, a homoeopathic remedy, an acupuncture treatment or anything else, you may still only be treating the symptom.

It is where side-effects outweigh benefits and when, because symptoms are being masked, we actually ignore underlying causes that we are heading for real trouble. There is no long-term benefit in masking the pain of an appendix that is about to burst – whether it is drugs, acupuncture, hydrotherapy or anything else that is doing the masking! There is nothing wrong, however, with treating symptoms *as long* as the underlying causes are *also* being addressed, and as long as the treatment being used is not creating more problems than it is solving.

## Removing causes

There are other ways of treating health problems and the most effective, where it is possible, is to remove the cause of whatever is happening. If someone has headaches because they need new prescription spectacles the 'cure' is obvious. If someone has indigestion because they eat junk food or because they don't chew adequately, the cure may also be obvious, but its application requires more discipline and effort on the part of the sufferer. In other words, knowing the cause does not always lead to appropriate action – the numbers of people who are new, or still, smokers are evidence enough of the truth of this.

### NON-SPECIFIC CONSTITUTIONAL METHODS

Yet another choice is available in terms of health promotion – to treat the body in a way that, instead of directing its aim at the symptoms makes its target the improvement of the efficiency of the self-repair mechanisms, encouraging homeostasis, a fully functioning immune system and so on.

The rationale behind this approach is simple: the body heals itself, while treatment never makes it do this. The most that treatment can ever achieve is an enhancement of the natural, innate, self-healing potentials of the body, either by removing obstacles to recovery or by assisting the mechanisms that repair and heal the body.

In the last chapter we saw two examples of such non-specific constitutional methods. The first was the practice of autogenic training, in which the mind is focused to reach a state of deep relaxation, similar to that achieved in deep meditation. This involves a quietening of mental activity, a calming of nervous system activity, a stilling of the chatter that usually dominates the mind, to reach a profoundly restful state in which brain wave patterns change, self-healing is amplified and negative activities (for example, a hyper-reactive sympathetic nervous system) are calmed or returned to normal functioning. So, the first of the constitutional methods recommended for anyone with chronic fatigue syndrome (ME) or fibromyalgia is a form of deep relaxation, and autogenic training is one of these.

In the section about detoxification in the previous chapter we came across the second – repetitive short-term fasting, which was suggested as a part of the process of detoxification. Fasting allows the body a period of physiological rest as there is no food to digest. There is ample evidence that this period of rest stimulates the self-healing mechanisms into action (Burton, Chaitow, 1993, 1987, Hoefel, 1928, Imamura, 1958, Kenton, 1988, Kernt, 1982, Keys, 1950, Kroker, 1983, Kjeldsen-Kragh, 1991, Mose, 1983, Weindruch and Walford, 1988, and Wing, 1983). Long fasts (those lasting weeks rather than days) cannot safely be undertaken at home without supervision, although these are even more effective than the repetitive short fasts described in Chapter 6, and so if anyone wishes to go through this remarkable regenerative process, they should do so in a clinic or spa that specializes in such procedures (Chaitow, 1994).

Fasting is a non-specific constitutional approach to healing and, as with deep relaxation, it has no absolutely clear-cut objectives, but is providing an opportunity for normal healing functions to operate more efficiently by offering a period of quiet, stillness, absence of the normal hustle of internal metabolic and digestive activity.

### A neutral bath

In the stress-reduction section of the previous chapter, the benefits of taking a neutral bath were described. This method provides an environment in which there is a profoundly reduced number of stimuli as the water in which you are immersed is at body heat. The stimulation of the peripheral neural structures is reduced and the constant factor of hydrostatic pressure on the body has a deeply relaxing physiological effect. This, too, is a constitutional, non-specific approach to healing and is highly recommended as a regular part of self-treatment for health promotion, especially if there is any tendency to anxiety, nervousness or sleep or pain problems.

In many centres, a neutral bath is now offered but they are called 'flotation tanks', in which the person is immersed in water of a neutral temperature, which has been saturated with Epsom and other salts, allowing you to float as though in the Dead Sea. Also, the tanks are enclosed and the lighting inside is very subdued, removing the stimuli of light and shapes (something easily achieved at home by wearing an eye mask), and 'white sound' music is played, which blocks out all other sound. The more stimuli that can be removed, whether they be those contacting the skin, temperature differentials, sound, light or others, the better as this helps achieve the state of calm stillness that allows healing to occur.

There remain two additional 'constitutional' methods to be described here (although there are many others), which are of major importance in the treatment of chronic fatigue and chronic pain conditions. The first involves progressive cold bathing (or showering).

The results of important hydrotherapy research in London involving 100 volunteers were published in *The European* (22 and

29 April 1993). The Thrombosis Research Institute (which conducted the research) claims that the use of this form of self-treatment proves without question the dramatic value of carefully graduated cold baths when taken regularly (daily for six months for optimal results).

The Institute, under the Director, Dr. Vijay Kakkar, has now gathered 5000 volunteers, many of them suffering from chronic fatigue syndrome (ME), for the next stage of this research into the benefits of what has been called 'thermo regulatory hydrotherapy' (TRH).

The results of the first study showed that, when applied correctly, the effect of TRH was:

- a boost to sex hormone production, which helps regulate both potency in men and fertility in women
- renewed energy – many chronic fatigue syndrome (ME) sufferers were found to improve dramatically and in one case, a person who had to spend 18 hours a day in bed due to their exhausted state, found 'a new lease of life' after treatment, the person concerned being quoted in *The European* as stating: 'From the first day I have regularly undertaken the hydrotherapy. With each day the feeling of well-being increases to such an extent that I can hardly wait for the next morning to arrive.'
- improved circulation in people with cold extremities – indeed, not only is the circulation found to improve rapidly with TRH, but levels of specific enzymes that help circulation rise
- reduced chances of heart attacks and strokes because of improved blood clotting function
- increased levels of white blood cells (defenders against infection)
- reduced levels of unpleasant menopausal symptoms
- some of the volunteers found that their nails became harder and their hair growth improved.

How was this achieved? There are four stages to TRH and it is essential to 'train' the body towards the beneficial response by going through these stages.

*Cautions:* When cold water treatments are used by people with fatigue problems, including ME, the degree of stimulus (that is, how cold the water is and how long the person is immersed) needs to be modified so that a very slow gradient of temperature change is achieved, gradually training and 'hardening' the body to what is potentially a stress factor.

To plunge someone who is extremely fragile in their ability to handle stress of any sort into cold water straight from the tap would be downright foolhardy, whereas taking a shower or bath in 'neutral' (body heat) water for a week before extremely gradually starting the process of, day by day, making the water used cooler and cooler, perhaps over a period of months before from-the-tap cold water is used, is both sensible and effective.

The TRH programme runs for 80 days and the degree of coldness and the length of time in the water is only gradually increased, so follow the method and even make the changes in temperature and length of time immersed more gradual if necessary.

*When not to use the method:* This cold water bath method is not recommended for people with well-established heart disease, high blood pressure or chronic diseases requiring regular prescription medication, unless a doctor has been consulted as to the use of TRH.

Studies in Germany have shown that repetitive daily cold showers produce, over a three – to six-month period, a marked enhancement of the immune system, with far fewer infections and the duration of those that do occur (colds or flu) being far shorter than in people having hot or warm showers.

PREPARATION
Have ready a bath, bath thermometer, watch and bath mat.

The bathroom needs to be at a reasonably comfortable temperature – not too cold and not very hot.

## METHOD

The temperature of the water should eventually be as it comes from the tap – cold. However, train yourself to accept the cold bath by first having a tepid bath for a few weeks, gradually making the water colder, so that it goes below body heat, until having a really cold bath is not a shock but is actually looked forward to because of the wonderful energy boost it gives.

The timings described below can also be modified so that, at first, the whole process takes just a few minutes as you pass through the various stages of immersion, with a slow increase in the length of time spent at each stage as well as a reduction in the temperature of the water.

- STAGE 1 Stand in the bath in cold water (the range recommended for this stage is between 12.7°C and 18.3°C, but take account of the cautions above and suit the coldness of the water to your degree of fragility/ robustness) for between 1 and 5 minutes. When you are fully used to the process, perhaps after some weeks, you can increase the time you spend in the water within this range as your internal thermostat (a part of the brain called the hypothalamus) starts to respond. Be sure to put the non-slip mat on the bottom of the bath and do not stand still but walk up and down the bath or march on the spot.
- STAGE 2 By now, your internal thermostat is primed and so you need to sit in the cold water for another 1 to 5 minutes – up to your waist ideally – so that the pooled blood in the lower half of the body is cooled and further influences the hypothalamus.

- STAGE 3 This is the most important part of the programme – immersing your body up to the neck and back of the head in the cold water. You need to gently and slowly move your arms and legs to ensure that the slightly warmer water touching the skin (warmed by you) is not static, so that the cooling effect continues. You can stay immersed like this for between 10 and 20 minutes when you are fully acclimatized, but you could stay in for as little as 2 minutes at first, always adjusting the degree of coldness according to your sensitivity.
- STAGE 4 This is the 'rewarming'. Get out of the bath, towel yourself dry and move around for a few minutes. As you warm up, a pleasant glowing sensation will be felt in various precise locations, such as the chest, feet and between the shoulder-blades.

The whole sequence (first standing, then sitting and finally lying down), modified by reducing time and increasing the water temperature at first as necessary (and only standing or standing and sitting in the first few weeks), needs to be done *every time and daily* if the training or 'hardening' effect is to be achieved – with some people finding that taking *several* cold baths daily improves their functioning and energy levels.

## NON-SPECIFIC BODYWORK

There is evidence that massage, applied regularly, repetitively and with progressive strength/intensity, can achieve similar 'hardening' effects (albeit more slowly than can hydrotherapy). Such an approach can be very useful in cases of chronic fatigue syndrome (ME) and fibromyalgia, as part of the methodology of treating muscular aches and pains in particular and fatigue in general.

The massage should be slow and rhythmical, non-specific, that is, not focused on trying to 'normalize' or 'do' anything, just repetitive and soothing. Gradually (week by week, not in any one treatment) the massage should be made deeper. In Chapters 8 and 9, a particular form of bodywork called strain-counterstrain will be outlined and explained. It is close to being a 'constitutional approach' to healing as it doesn't force change, but, rather, allows it to happen.

## ACUPUNCTURE

In acupuncture, there is a distinction between treating the patient's symptoms and offering a balancing and harmonizing approach that aims to restore equilibrium to the energy flows of the body. This, too, is a 'constitutional' treatment as it makes no pretence at focusing on anything other than restoring general balance and allows that desirable state to provide the opportunity for other dysfunctions to normalize themselves.

### Two other manual methods

Very light massage, using manual lymphatic drainage – 5 times a week for 3 weeks – has been shown to be a safe and valuable treatment in reducing pain and enhancing the quality of life for fibromyalgia patients (Ekici *et al.*, 2009).

In another research study 70 patients with a diagnosis of fibromyalgia – average age 57 – received 10 treatments with a device that delivered deep oscillation massage – twice weekly over a period of five weeks. After this period symptoms were improved significantly. It is thought that the deep vibration causes release in the tissues of nitric oxide which has a relaxing effect and enhances circulation (Kraft *et al.*, 2011).

### A final thought

We should consider these approaches – the appropriate use of hydrotherapy, bodywork and acupuncture – as modulating or balancing rather than 'boosting' immune function and in this way enhancing homeostasis and so acting constitutionally as do deep relaxation, fasting and neutral baths.

# 8

# Manual Methods for Fibromyalgia and Myofascial Pain Syndrome

Pain relief depends on appropriate intervention. This often calls for multidimensional approaches that may act in one of a number of ways to interrupt the transmission of pain impulses – for example, by stimulating the production of the body's own painkilling substances, by altering the person's perception of the pain, by removal of the factors that are causing or perpetuating the pain, by normalizing structural imbalances or chemical factors that might be involved, by altering energy factors or by any combination of these influences.

As will become clear from the evidence in the next chapter, the most successful manipulative methods in treating fibromyalgia have been derived from osteopathic methodology. The truth is that, in recent years, the differences between the methods used by qualified osteopaths, chiropractors and physiotherapists have reduced. Indeed, they increasingly use similar manipulation methods to each other to help mobilize and normalize restricted areas.

A number of reports of studies mentioned in the orthodox medical press have shown the superiority of osteopathic and chiropractic methods in dealing with back and neck pain problems compared with standard medical care given for these troublesome complaints.

Help is also frequently available from massage therapists who use a wide variety of soft tissue techniques, many of which are identical to those used by osteopaths.

## Seek a diagnosis before you have any treatment

It is essential when treating muscular and joint dysfunction that a sound assessment is made as to the locations of joint and muscular restrictions, tender and trigger points, as well as of overall structural and postural integrity (soundness, that is whether or not there is balance and so on). It is also vital that treatment takes account of the potential causes (and aggravating factors) of the pain, whether this involves emotional distress, postural imbalances or functional factors, including breathing problems, such as asthma, bronchitis or hyperventilation.

Biochemical, hormonal, nutritional, toxic and other elements can also be associated with musculoskeletal dysfunction, as we have seen in earlier chapters, and if this is the case, it is obvious that the treatment methods of choice will involve efforts to normalize these imbalances. Just because a pain is in a muscle does not mean that it is the muscle that should be the focus of attention!

## Empowerment and awareness

It is also extremely important where pain is concerned that the person suffering the pain understands, as far as is possible, what the mechanisms of the situation are – the causes and processes of the condition – and the aims and likely effects of any treatment.

Along with understanding the processes involved in their chronic pain and its treatment, the patient needs to develop some means of exercising control over it, even if this is of a temporary nature. It may not always be possible to eliminate all symptoms, whichever approaches are adopted, but it should always be possible to moderate, modulate or in some way alter the intensity, duration and type of discomfort and pain being endured.

An enormous amount of research into chronic pain in particular and chronic illness in general has shown that these two factors – understanding and control – are the keys to learning to cope with the condition.

One element that also always needs to be incorporated, however difficult, is that of constructive self-treatment.

*Caution:* Before you use any self-help measures for chronic problems, make sure you receive a diagnosis and professional advice and/or treatment as well.

There are a number of safe and effective self-help body-work methods derived from osteopathic and other disciplines that can be used in cases of pain, strain and stiffness, whether it is for chronic pain or as first aid in acute episodes.

### Strain-counterstrain methods

One of the most successful approaches to treating pain is called strain-counterstrain and it derives from osteopathic practice.

In the case of almost any painful condition – acute or chronic – apply the following simple methods and you may well be amazed at the relief you get from them (even if this is only short-lived if the underlying causes have not been eliminated).

METHOD

- Gently test the area (muscle, joint) to see which precise movements cause you discomfort or pain or are restricted, carefully noting in which direction pain or restriction exists or is produced. For example, it might hurt you most to turn your neck to the right and look upwards (or there could be restriction in moving in these directions) while turning left and looking down might hurt less or not at all and may be free of restriction. What you are doing is noting which directions of movement are restricted or painful, not where the pain is felt.

- Search, by means of gentle finger or thumb pressure, for tender or sore points in the soft tissues (muscles, ligaments and so on) that would be working if the *opposite* movement to that which caused you pain was being performed. In the example given above, these would be the muscles on the left and front of your neck, which are the muscles that would help your head to turn to the *left* and bend *forwards* (because it hurt to turn *right* and tilt *upwards*).

- Once you have found the most tender point in these muscles, keep a light pressure on it so that you can use it to guide you in the next stage of the method.

- Now, very gently and slowly, move the area (in the example we have been using, your head and neck) until you find a position in which the tenderness goes out of the point on which you are lightly pressing.

- Any movement that causes you increased pain (either in the neck or head in our example) or on that point is in the wrong direction. You will find that there is always a position of 'maximum ease' in which both the neck and head in this example and the tender point will be either pain free or far less uncomfortable (see Figure 8.1, page 184).

- You have to find that position yourself, but, generally, if the tender point is on the front of your body, you will probably have to bend forwards to ease it, as well as bending to the side of the pain and rotating towards it in most cases, whereas if the tender point is on the back of the body, you may have to bend backwards and make additional 'fine-tuning' movements, which may include twisting or bending away from the side of the pain, in order to manipulate the tissues into a (relatively) pain-free state. Remember that the objective of your efforts

**Figure 8.1** *Careful positioning of the head and neck removes sensitivity from the tender point that is being pressed. This helps to find a position of ease, which is held while the muscles relax. After this, the neck will be freer than before and usually less painful.*

is that of taking the tenderness out of the spot on which you are pressing, but, whatever movements this calls for, pain should not increase in the affected area (the neck and head in our example) or create new pain anywhere else.

■ In the example, where it is painful to turn your head right and look up, you would search for the tender point in the muscles on the left and front of your neck and upper shoulder area, which would need to be active to produce the exact opposite movement. Having found a suitably tender point and while holding light pressure on it (enough to cause mild pain), you would probably find that by letting your head tilt forwards and down, with a little turn to the left and possibly bending to one side or the other, while possibly slightly lifting your left shoulder, the pain would vanish from the point. To do this you might need to be lying down so that the area is supported, which it would not be if you were sitting or standing.

- Once you have found the position of ease, rest there for at *least* a minute before slowly returning to a neutral position (back to where you started). The whole area should now feel easier and less painful and restricted, and the movement that produced pain before should do so to a far lesser degree. Also, the tender point should be far less irritable on pressure than before.

You can use this method for any recent strain, sprain or restriction or for any painful point you locate. You can also use this strain-counterstrain method, exactly as described above, on any tender or sore point in any muscle in the body. If the pain is chronic, the relief may only be short-lived, but if it has only come on recently, the relief can be permanent.

In the next chapter, you will find guidelines as to how to treat sensitivity and pain in the first five of the points used to diagnose fibromyalgia (this makes ten points altogether as there is always a corresponding point on each side of the body). Practice finding these to see how you can use the strain-counterstrain method to normalize or ease these pain points, but don't forget to seek tender points in 'opposite' muscles when a movement hurts or is restricted.

It is worth re-emphasizing that the strain-counterstrain technique will reduce pain and restriction to some extent in most chronic pain problems, but the results may not last very long as fibrotic changes will probably have taken place in the soft tissues (see Chapter 4), requiring additional treatment (such as muscle energy treatment, described below) from a professional.

## HOW DOES THIS POSITIONAL RELEASE METHOD WORK?

What seems to be happening, according to research, is that when a stressed area of muscle is placed in a position of ease, nerve reporting stations (called muscle spindles) reset themselves and so reduce the amount of excessive tension or tone that the muscle is holding (Chaitow, 1989, Jones, 1981). If the muscle was previously in spasm, or even just being held in a state of tension, this would relax and free the tissues, at least for a time.

Additional research has shown that when in a position of ease, muscles enjoy a greatly improved blood supply. This means that if the muscle had been relatively short of oxygen before being positioned in this way, it would, after the experience, be better oxygenated and nourished and should therefore be less painful (Rathbun and Macnab, 1970).

Much of the success of the method depends on how long the position of ease is held, which indicates that something is actually happening during that time other than simply being in a relatively pain-free position. The benefit, as we have seen, seems to stem from a combination of a neural resetting of tone and improved circulation.

All this relates to the final message of the previous chapter in that strain-counterstrain fits into the 'constitutional' approach to healing – it does not 'make' anything happen, but provides a space in which self-normalization processes can operate, just as deep relaxation, fasting and neutral baths do.

### Muscle energy treatment and self-treatment for muscles and joints

There are two powerful built-in methods (Baldry, 1993, Brodin, 1987, Chaitow, 1989, Janda, 1992, Lewit, 1992, Simons, 1985) that you can use to safely release tight and tense muscles or to deactivate trigger points, which are often a cause of continuing pain and stiffness:

- post-isometric relaxation
- reciprocal inhibition.

## POST-ISOMETRIC RELAXATION

When a muscle has been contracted for seven seconds or more without being able to actually move (known as an isometric exercise or contraction), the muscle will be far more pliable and easy to stretch afterwards than it was before the contraction. This effect is a normal physiological one that we can use to help free and stretch tight, painful tissues very gently.

## RECIPROCAL INHIBITION

When a muscle is contracted isometrically (that is, it is contracted and not allowed to move), it causes its opposing muscle to relax, allowing it to be stretched more easily and painlessly after the contraction (the muscle that opposes another one is known as its antagonist, and every muscle has antagonists or we would only be able to move ourselves in one direction and not back again).

## USING THESE PRINCIPLES

From the above, we know that when a muscle can be contracted against an unyielding resistance, the muscle and its antagonist will be more relaxed (see Figure 8.2, page 188). For example, if turning your head to the right is difficult and painful, this could be because the muscles on the left of the neck are tense and tight, preventing easy movement away from that side. You could try to turn your head to the left against resistance, provided by your own hands, achieving this perhaps by sitting at a table with your head resting in your hands. As you try to turn your head to the left against the resistance of your hand, you will be contracting the very muscles that are preventing you easily turning your head to the right. After a 10-second contraction, using only about 20 per cent of your strength to make the turning movement, you should (because of post-isometric relaxation) be able to turn your head

**Figure 8.2** *By contracting a tense muscle against unmoving resistance for seven to ten seconds, post-isometric relaxation occurs, which eases the tension in that muscle. The antagonist muscle will also be relaxed by this contraction because of reciprocal inhibition. Both mechanisms are part of muscle energy technique (MET).*

to the right more easily and painlessly. This is because the muscles on the left will have been forced to relax painlessly.

Alternatively, you could use the principle of reciprocal inhibition. Using the same situation as above, try resisting your attempt to turn your head to the right (as long as the effort is not painful). This would use the antagonists of the muscles, which are probably short (on the left side) and which are preventing easy movement to the right.

After the contraction is over (hold the position for 10 seconds or so) there would have been inhibition of the muscles on the left and so it should be easier to turn to the right.

Even if you have no obvious problem, try this method. Sit at a table, rest your head on your hands and try to release tightness in the neck muscles and so increase the range of rotation. We all have enough tension in our necks to demonstrate the improvement these simple methods can produce (see Figure 8.3).

**Figure 8.3** *Muscle energy technique being applied to a stiff neck to ease excessive tension (tonicity) of the muscles.*

## GUIDELINES

- Never use more than 20 per cent of the strength in the muscles when using either post-isometric relaxation or reciprocal inhibition.
- Never produce pain when doing these exercises. If you do, you are either using too much effort or you should switch to working on the antagonist muscles as the ones you are using are too sensitive.
- After the contraction, wait a few seconds until you have relaxed and then gently stretch the muscles a little further than they could go before the contraction.
- Repeat the process as often as you like, as long as no pain is produced and as long as you are finding you are able to stretch further each time.
- You will get better results from post-isometric relaxation than reciprocal inhibition, but may have to use this latter method if post-isometric relaxation is painful.

You can use these muscle energy methods to treat any stiff or painful area to release tension or to totally or partially switch off trigger point activity in the muscles, as often as you wish, whether the restriction or stiffness is a muscle or a joint (the movements of all joints are governed by muscles). Even an arthritic joint can be made more flexible by these methods, if only for a short time, as long as you stick precisely to the method and guidelines (Chaitow, 1989, Baldry, 1993, Janda, 1992, Lewit, 1992) given above.

*When should you choose strain-counterstrain methods and when muscle energy treatment?*
Strain-counterstrain is best for acute problems and is ideal if muscle spasms are associated with it (lumbago and wry neck are two good examples of such conditions).

It is probably the least invasive bodywork approach and so is ideal for those in a lot of pain who are very sensitive or do not need the additional stress of painful treatment.

Muscle energy treatment is best where there is restriction, stiffness and a limited range of movement, with or without painful associations, and as trigger points (those points that are painful and refer symptoms) have to be stretched to normalize their activity, this form of treatment is the obvious and safest way of deactivating these noxious pain centres.

Either or both methods can be used on any given pain or stiffness problem, to ease spasm and pain and increase the range of movement.

Using strain-counterstrain followed by muscle energy treatment is thought to be a most effective way of reducing trigger point activity in myofascial pain syndrome, but they need to be performed by a professional bodywork expert (Chaitow, 1989). Indeed, self-treatment using muscle energy treatment methods should not replace professional advice, unless complete relief is achieved after using them just once or twice as first aid. They are ideal methods to use as first aid and to support what is being done by skilled healthcare professionals.

## Finding and treating trigger points

Many people suffer years of pain, such as chronic headaches, and it has nothing to do with the area in which they feel the pain because it is, in fact, being exported there from somewhere else – from one or more trigger points.

To refresh your memory on the description of trigger points given in Chapter 4, they occur when, due to mechanical and other forms of stress, certain muscular areas of the body become 'facilitated', which means extremely easily irritated. When this happens, the nerve impulses that pass through or derive from them become increasingly sensitive and capable of causing quite severe pain in distant 'target' areas. Examples of common triggers and targets include head pain that comes from triggers in the neck and shoulder muscles; abdominal pain that comes from triggers in the back; breast pain that comes from arm muscle triggers; knee pain that comes from triggers in the thigh and foot; and toe pains that come from triggers in the shin area.

There are many pain patterns (see the list below) that can be successfully treated using either painkilling injections, acupuncture, acupressure, chilling techniques (cryotherapy), soft tissue manipulation techniques (muscle energy treatment and strain-counterstrain techniques), electrotherapy and others, some of which (mainly pressure and stretching techniques) you can use to treat yourself.

*When should you suspect that your pain results from myofascial pain syndrome?*
If your pain has no obvious cause, such as a joint strain or an arthritic condition, say, and seems persistent, despite treatment or rest or after you have had treatment for a problem that was supposed to be the cause, you might start suspecting that you have myofascial pain syndrome. Be especially suspicious of trigger point activity if your pain is worse when you are under different forms of stress, say after physical effort or emotional upset or a chill or

any other form of stress, especially if the stress does not directly involve the area of pain.

### How to find trigger points

- If you carefully search muscles that are sensitive or tight with your fingers, you will find very sensitive local areas of muscle that seem more fibrous, stringy or even slightly swollen (the skin overlying these points will often have a characteristic 'rough' feel when you stroke it very lightly), and when you press such an area, this causes a new pain to appear some distance away. The new pain is in what is called a target area, and this might well be a place where you have been feeling pain for some time (see Figure 8.4 for an example).

- If you have a recurrent ache or pain in a part of your body (your head, face, back, hips or other part) that does not seem to worsen when you press carefully with your fingers on the area or seems to have no obvious cause, then use the trigger point maps (see page 196) and information to see

**Figure 8.4** *A trigger point, when active (or when pressed), will refer pain and other symptoms (sometimes numbness, sometimes pins and needles, etc.) to a target area. This is a facilitated area and any stress affecting the person as a whole will also irritate the trigger point.*

whether or not these might themselves be target areas, by working backwards from the target to where the trigger for that target is usually found.

■ Search this area with a finger or thumb until you find a discrete, localized contraction, a grain-like structure or 'swelling'. Press this and see if you can't, in fact, reproduce the pain in the target area. If you can, you have found the trigger point and need to treat it or have it treated professionally by a therapist.

■ In inaccessible areas where your hands cannot easily reach (your lower back, for example) use a tennis ball to apply the pressure. Lie on a carpet and place the ball under your back and roll around on it carefully, letting your weight on the ball increase whenever you want to press a particular place. You can give yourself an effective massage of the area in this way as well as uncovering the presence of triggers. You can also place two balls inside an old sock, tie the top and use the balls to massage your spine by lying on them, positioning one ball each side of the spine. By gently moving up and down, you can roll on the balls, allowing them to release muscle tension by pressure.

## Trigger point patterns

■ Trigger points found along the upper surface and top, inner angle of the shoulder-blades refer pain to the head, face, neck and shoulders.

■ The border of the shoulder-blade near the spine or its lower angle refers to target areas in the upper arms and to the little finger-side of the hand; sometimes to the front of the shoulders.

■ Trigger points in the upper trapezius (this is the muscle running from the base of the skull to the shoulder) refer pain to the area behind the ear or the forehead. Search this muscle by gently squeezing or pinching it rather than pressure.

- Trigger points on the upper surface of the sacral bone (base of the spine) are involved in many pain problems in the back and pelvic regions.
- Lower back pain is also associated with trigger points on the outer border of the large muscles near the spine at waist level (quadratus lumborum). Pressure to reach trigger points here needs to be from the side of the muscle, not from the back.
- Sometimes pressure here accesses trigger points in the muscle that runs from the pelvis to the arm up the back and side (latissimus dorsi), which will refer pain to the shoulder or arm.
- The muscles of the buttocks (glutei) carry trigger points, especially just under the rim of the pelvic bones, which can send pain to the hips, down the leg (back usually) and outer foot.
- Pain down the leg that mimics sciatic pain is also caused by triggers in the piriformis muscle, which can lie either just behind the hip joint or a little further back towards the sacrum.
- Trigger points lying on the back of the leg, about 10 cm (4 in) above the knee refer pain to the knee and calf.
- Lower calf pain can also result from a trigger point that lies just below the broadest part of the calf, in the gastrocnemius muscle, or lower in the calf, in the soleus muscle.
- Trigger points in the neck muscles can refer pain to the shoulders or the head and face. Search for trigger points by gently squeezing the muscle that runs from the breastbone and collar-bone to behind the ear (sternomastoid) up to the bone behind the ear (mastoid), working up from where the muscle inserts into the collar-bone (central and midline part), and the upper surface of the breastbone, where trigger points refer pain to the face and head.
- In the same area of the side and front of the neck lie the

scalene muscles, which house trigger points that refer pain to the arm and hand (squeeze them rather than pressing).

- Trigger points that are found in the jaw muscles refer to the tempero-mandibular joint and can be a cause of tinnitus and eye problems.
- Trigger points in the pectoral muscles and just below the collar-bone can refer pain to the arm or into the chest or down the side of the body (see Figure 8.4).
- Trigger points that lie in the small muscles between the ribs can refer pain to the chest, back or internally.
- The large bicep muscle in the upper arm inserts into the arm by a tendon and in this area trigger points are found that refer pain to the shoulder.
- On the breastbone (sternum) itself, there is very little muscle and yet trigger points can be found that refer across the chest to either shoulder or both.
- Abdominal muscle trigger points can refer to the sides, downwards or up towards the chest.
- Trigger points on the inner thigh refer to the hip or down the leg to the knee.
- Trigger points in the muscles of the side of the thigh (tensor fascia lata) produce sciatic-type pain.
- Trigger points in the front of the lower leg refer to the foot and ankle.

These examples represent the major trigger points (see Figure 8.5, page 196), but there are hundreds of possibilities.

## TREATING TRIGGER POINTS

There are many ways in which to successfully treat trigger points yourself. It is more likely though, if the pain of myofascial pain syndrome is chronic, that you will need professional help. What follows can be used alone to treat a new or not too intense pain or as an adjunct to treatment received from your healthcare professional.

**Figure 8.5** *These are some of the major trigger points. They occur in areas that are commonly stressed by overuse and postural faults. Pressure on the trigger point will produce pain both in it and the target area, while pressure on the target area normally feels like pressure, without pain.*

Trigger point in levator scapula muscle refers
pain to shoulder blade, shoulder and neck.

Supraspinatus muscle trigger point refers pain
to the outer aspect of the arm, front and back.

Gluteus minimus trigger point refers pain in
the buttock, the posterior and lateral thigh, and calf.

Hamstring (biceps femoris) muscle trigger point refers pain
to the back of the of the lower thigh and knee.

Gastrocnemius muscle trigger point refers pain
to the calf, ankle and sole of the foot.

Posterior cervical muscle trigger point refers pain
to the base of the skull, the neck and shoulder blade.

a) Sternomastoid muscle trigger point refers to pain to the side
and front of the neck as well as to the head and jaw.
b) Pressure on this should be squeezing rather than pushing,
as there are sensitive structures underneath it.

Temporalis muscle trigger point refers pain to
the side of the head but more strongly to the
area above the eyes, and the teeth and mouth.

Pectoralis muscle trigger point refers pain to the
chest and inner arm, especially around the elbow.

Serratus anterior trigger point refers pain to
the side of the upper ribs, down the arm to the
hand and to the lower part of the shoulder blade.

Deltoid muscle trigger point refers pain to
the shoulder and side and front of the upper arm.

Sternalis muscle trigger point refers pain to
the breast bone, towards the throat and across
both sides of the chest to the shoulders.

Upper trapezius muscle trigger point refers
pain to the neck, head and temple area.

Lower multifidus muscle trigger point refers
pain to the lower ribs, the lower spinal areas and
to the lower abdomen on the same side.

Adductor longus trigger point refers pain
to the groin, front of leg and inner knee.

Long extensor muscle trigger point refers pain
to the shin, outer foot and toes.

The trigger point needs to be deactivated to some extent, and you can do this by using direct finger, thumb or tennis ball pressure in the following way:

- first, use enough pressure that you can just feel the pain in the target area and maintain this pressure for about 7 to 10 seconds before easing off, not letting go of the place, but not applying any pressure for a further 5 seconds
- repeat this process of 10 seconds (or so) pressure followed by 5 seconds rest for up to 2 minutes (but do not go over a total of 8 full cycles of on and off pressure)
- alternatively, stop just as soon as the referred (target area) pain feels as if it is lessening.

Instead of this pressure method, you can try to start deactivating the trigger point by using the strain-counterstrain method described above. After either two minutes of pressure or at least a minute of 'ease' in the appropriate counterstrain position, you need to move to the next stage of the self-treatment.

The next stage is to stretch the muscles in which the trigger point is sited, and you can try using muscle energy treatment (as described above) to do this if the muscle is in a suitable place (it is very hard to stretch muscles between your shoulder blades yourself, for example, but quite easy to stretch muscles between the neck and shoulder – a common trigger point area). Unfortunately, unless the muscles in which trigger points lie are stretched after treatment, the trigger will very soon become active again. So, stretching is a must.

Ideally, of course, you should be having the treatment done for you by a skilled therapist, but if this is not possible, try the following.

- If possible, during the stretching, you should chill the muscle in which the trigger point lies. One good way of doing this is to roll (for no more than about 20 seconds in any one minute) a cold metallic object over the muscle, running it in slow sweeps from the trigger point towards the target area. The easiest way to provide such chilling is to fill an empty soft drink can with water and freeze it. When treating the area as described, take care to keep it moving.

■ So, you apply pressure, stretch and chill the muscle (doing the last two at the same time) and this will usually start the process of deactivating trigger point activity. All other forms of treatment for trigger points should be professionally administered (injections, acupuncture and so on).

■ After treating the trigger point, rest the whole area for a day or so, avoiding any strenuous movements. Immediately after the treatment, placing a damp, hot towel (rung out in hot water) over the treated point for 15 minutes is helpful and soothing.

### Self-massage for pain relief

*Cautions:* Do not give yourself or any one else a massage if there is a current health problem unless you have professional approval or instruction. Particularly:

■ avoid tissues that are actively inflamed or where blood vessels are inflamed

■ avoid massaging where active infection is present

■ avoid massaging if there is a heart condition, unless professional advice supports doing so

■ avoid massage if there is a cancerous condition – although there is evidence that it can be of benefit (as a way of reducing stress) when it is performed under professional guidance (Weinrech, 1990)

■ avoid massage if there has been haemorrhage or other causes of bleeding in the tissues

■ do not massage in the area of a recent fracture or sprain.

Two key features help maintain pain when muscles are tense and tight:

- an inadequate supply of fresh, oxygenated blood
- the retention, congestion or build-up of waste products in the tissues.

Massage can very successfully help normalize both these features, even if this is only for a short time. Massage also produces relaxation and a reduction in anxiety levels (especially when skilfully performed) and, to some extent, self-massage can achieve this, too.

Self-massage, or massage performed by a partner or family member, can be very effective if the strokes are applied rhythmically in a systematic manner – although nothing can compare with the treatment received from a professionally trained massage therapist.

The following techniques are easily learned for use at home. Note that massage should never hurt and should be performed slowly and rhythmically.

## EFFLEURAGE

*Preparation*
Apply a massage cream or oil gently to the skin over the area to be massaged so that you will not drag the skin when you are massaging.

*Method*

- Make the first strokes slow, long ones, using the heels of the hands, the palms of the hands or the thumbs. Keep your hands relaxed but firm and mould them to the shapes and contours of the area you are working on.

- As you massage the area, no pain should be produced and the pressure applied should match the sensitivity of the area.
- Ideally, as one hand is moving forwards over the area, the other should be coming back, so an alternating, rhythmic series of pleasant stroking actions soothes the region. Often a circular action is appropriate, so one hand is following the other in slow, pleasing circles.
- On a large area, such as the thigh, stroke away from you with the heel of the hand for a distance of about 30.5 cm (12 in) and then circle back again. As the hand is slowly returning towards you, let the other commence its stroke. You are now doing effleurage!
- Continue with these movements for several minutes, varying the area you are working on slightly after a few repetitions. Use a similar pattern again after some of the other methods described below and, perhaps, finish the whole session with stroking as well.

Traditionally, effleurage is performed with the stroke moving towards the heart (up the leg, for example). This is not always easy when massaging parts of yourself, however, and perhaps it is more important in these circumstances to remember the guidelines not to cause pain and to try to achieve a feeling of relaxation of the tissues.

## PETRISSAGE
This involves a kneading, wringing action in which muscles are held and lifted by one hand and then the other. One hand grasps a handful of muscle firmly but gently, lifting and pulling it towards you, while the other pushes the adjacent tissue away from you, producing a kneading, squeezing and wringing movement.

*Preparation*
As for effleurage.

*Method*

- Start by pressing downwards with the heel of one hand while you lift the tissue with the fingers and thumb of that hand. Lift and gently squeeze or roll the handful of muscle before letting the other hand take over and do the same.
- Repeat this process, of one hand releasing its grip as the other takes over (just like kneading bread dough), rhythmically several times before moving to another part of the muscle.
- In some areas, two hands can work simultaneously, lifting, wringing and twisting the tissues. They can either perform the same actions or one can lift and push in one direction while the other lifts and pulls adjacent tissue, causing no pain, but creating light stretching.

## TAPPING

Tapping and vibrating tissues can produce a very relaxing effect and reduce pain sensations markedly.

*Preparation*

Before shaking the tissues (see Method), take hold of them firmly, but not painfully.

*Method*

- Try shaking the tissues gently, getting a vibration effect. Continue for a minute and then move to another area close by.
- Alternatively, with the side of the hand, make a series of chopping actions towards the muscle so that the fingertips (keep them relaxed) strike the muscle like drumsticks hitting a drum. By doing this lightly, quickly and repetitively (called tapotement), a very pleasing sensation can be created.

## THUMB WORK

Wherever you feel local tension in the muscles or bands of tight, tense tissue, use the thumbs or the heel of your hand to push across or into the area, taking out the slack – never causing pain, but pressing sufficiently hard to produce a 'nice hurt'. Hold such pressure for up to 10 seconds at a time before moving on or applying a gentle effleurage to soothe it.

## TENNIS BALL MASSAGE

Some areas are hard to reach, such as the lower back, and you may need to massage yourself here. If your partner or a friend is not available, try the following.

- Place a tennis ball on the carpet and lie on it so that it presses in the area of muscular pain you want to work on.
- Gently move yourself over it so that it presses and pushes the muscle until you feel easier.
- Try using a squash or golf ball to achieve a similar effect for the soles of the feet.

### Exercises to use in the treatment of fibromyalgia and muscle pain

Well-chosen exercises can be very helpful in most rehabilitation programmes where pain is a feature of musculoskeletal problems. There is now ample evidence that in fibromyalgia, often cardiovascular (aerobic) training produces a great improvement (McCain, 1986). You need to start with very mild degrees of effort and slowly increase the amount you do as your tolerance of it improves (see also Chapter 10).

It is essential to ensure that exercises do not make matters worse and, ideally, that things improve. An exercise programme should therefore be chosen and taught by a skilled health professional, who can work out precisely just how high your pulse rate can be safely and usefully taken during exercise of this sort.

Because of the very individual nature of exercise and rehabilitation programmes, it is almost impossible to give guidelines here, except very general ones.

## SOME GUIDELINES

Stretching (yoga, T'ai chi or muscle energy-type releases are safest) and movement in water are the ideal forms of stretching self-help and therapy. Most people with fibromyalgia will feel stiff some of the time, some feeling stiff most of the time. Flexibility can be regained to a degree, sometimes completely, by regular, painless, focused stretching and stretching movements.

Regarding aerobics, any safe movement that does not produce pain is suitable, and this could involve anything from skipping, to brisk walking or dancing. Rebound (trampoline) exercise is also effective, as is cycling and pool work or swimming. The level of aerobic exercise (cardiovascular training) that is optimal for fibromyalgia sufferers seems to involve employing enough effort to achieve between 75 and 85 per cent of your own safe heart rate potential (this needs to be calculated for you and, ideally, the figure arrived at should be based on your age and resting pulse rate) and maintain it for 20 minutes at least, 3 times a week. The objective is to ensure a more efficient delivery of adequately oxygenated blood to the tissues. Always start any new programme of exercise slowly, especially if you are unaccustomed to taking exercise – it is a training process and you must ensure that you do not do too much too soon.

If you have chronic fatigue syndrome (ME) and muscular pain, you probably find this suggestion to take aerobic exercise laughable. You are thinking that the usually simple task of getting dressed in the morning requires all your available energy, never mind active exercise. However, many people with such conditions or fibromyalgia can do aerobic exercise and it is to these individuals that these suggestions are directed. Remember, though, that fast, repetitive exercises or movements are more likely to be irritating to pain conditions than are slowly performed stretching movements. If it is possible for you to take part in active aerobic exercises without increasing the amount of pain you experience or irritating existing conditions (take advice on this), it is well established that such activity reduces stress levels, reduces anxiety and some natural painkilling substances are released by the body as a result.

In any given painful condition, if you move the affected area or other parts of the body very carefully in all possible directions, some movements will be more and some will be less painful than others. You can use muscle energy treatment (post-isometric relaxation and reciprocal inhibition) methods or those of strain-counterstrain (see the next chapter as well) to increase your pain-free range before doing such an assessment. If you can identify which movements cause no increase in pain at the time they are performed or afterwards, you can begin to build up a sequence of simple exercises (in water or at home) that will help maintain muscle tone and circulation. For example, you may find that it is painless to move your arm in one or two directions, but painful to move it in others. Slowly, take it in the painless directions a number of times, several times daily, in order to keep muscles toned and the circulation active. If actual movement is too painful, just tensing and relaxing the various muscles of the area can do a lot of good as this results in a 'pumping' of blood and lymph and maintains some degree of muscle 'fitness'. After doing whatever pain-free exercises you can several times a day (never allowing them to increase your pain levels), you can retest the direction and range of pain-free motion after a week or so and introduce any new pain-free movements that you may then be able to do, extending the range of movement.

If the pain is too great to allow the area to be moved, then see whether movements of areas distant to it will allow you to help the circulation and muscle tone of the affected area. For example,

---

if the lower back is too painful to move in any direction, then arm and leg movements that don't hurt the back can be useful.

There is growing evidence that just *thinking* about a particular movement slightly activates the muscles that would perform that action (Chaitow, 1989, Baldry, 1993, Lewit, 1992). So it can help to simply visualize particular movements, even if they cannot be performed because of pain.

Similarly, eye movements activate muscles in the direction in which the eyes are moving. If you look upwards with your eyes (not necessarily the neck and head as well), the muscles that are involved when you bend your neck and back backwards will increase in tone in preparation for that movement. So, by doing slow and deliberate eye movements, it is possible to give some exercise to the main muscles of the body.

Be very cautious about trying to strengthen what appears to be weak muscles. For example, it is often advocated that abdominal muscle weakness should be dealt with by doing sit-up-type exercises. The truth is that there is research and clinical (rehabilitation) evidence to show that such exercises often make matters worse. Why should this be? Weakness in one muscle or group of muscles is often the direct result of inhibitory (weakening) messages coming from the antagonists of the weak muscles. In the case of the abdominals, the weakening messages usually come from very tight lower back muscles and the way to efficiently and permanently restore strength to the weak abdominals is by relaxing and stretching the tight and short lower back muscles. When the tight lower back is ignored and exercises are done to tone weak abdominals, what usually happens is that the tight muscles get tighter and the weak ones weaker. General movement in water or walking will help to maintain tone and is safer than trying to 'strengthen' what appear to be weak muscles but which are in reality inhibited ones (Jull and Janda, 1987).

In the case of hypermobile joints (which are common in children with fibromyalgia), there may be general exercises that can be done to help increase balance and tone, such as swimming. This is a far safer approach than trying to build up muscle tone in joint areas to compensate for lax ligaments. Also, with any joint problems – ankles, knees, hips or back – put cushioned insoles into shoes or wear well-padded trainers. The reduction in the amount of shock absorbing the joints have to cope with by making such a simple change can be quite astounding. The amount of stress weight-bearing joints are subjected to can be reduced by up to half in this way.

**What we can learn from research on exercise and fibromyalgia**

When women with fibromyalgia were asked to perform different forms of exercise – aerobic, or aerobic combined with strength and conditioning, twice a week (45 to 60 minutes each time) for 24 weeks – both groups responded well. They demonstrated significantly less pain, increased vitality and mental health, as well as improved range.

# 9

# Strain-Counterstrain Treatment for Some Tender Points in Fibromyalgia

This chapter will help you to learn to use strain-counterstrain methods by focusing on some of the key tender points experienced by those with fibromyalgia. Not all the points can be worked on easily in self-treatment and so only those you can treat yourself are discussed.

What should emerge when you follow the guidelines is a sense of being able to treat your own pain by this simple, non-invasive method a method that is commonly used by osteopaths to treat pain, including that associated with fibromyalgia (see the next chapter).

Once you have practised the methods given in this chapter, you should be able to use strain-counterstrain methods to treat any painful point you happen to find, using the rules safely and effectively, whenever you wish.

### The locations of the tender points

You will recall from Chapter 1 that in order to be diagnosed as having fibromyalgia, at least 11 out of 18 points tested using a set amount of pressure (not more than 4 kg/8¼ lbs).

These 18 points lie in 9 sites each side of the body, and in this chapter the strain-counterstrain methods most likely to modify their tenderness will be described for the first 5 of these, enabling you to treat 10 sites.

The tender points tested to give a diagnosis of fibromyalgia are located in the following sites:

- either side of the base of the skull where the suboccipital muscles insert
- either side of the side of the neck, between the fifth and seventh cervical vertebrae
- either side of the body on the midpoint of the muscle that runs from the neck to the shoulder (the upper trapezius)
- either side of the body, where the supraspinatus muscle runs along the upper border of the shoulder-blade
- either side, on the upper surface of the rib, where the second rib meets the breastbone, in the pectoral muscle
- on the outer aspect of either elbow, just below the part that sticks out (epicondyle)
- in the large buttock muscles, either side, on the upper, outer aspect, in the fold in front of the muscle (gluteus medius)
- just behind the large bump you can feel of either hip joint where the piriformis muscle inserts
- on either knee in the fatty pad just above the inner aspect of the joint.

Additional sites sometimes also recommended for testing are:

- the lower portion of the sternomastoid muscle at the front of the body on the throat
- the lateral part of the pectoral muscle at the level of the fourth rib
- the region of the lower end of the spine, around the fourth and fifth lumbar vertebrae.

Let us now see how to treat the first five tender points given above.

---

### Treating tender points

SUBOCCIPITAL MUSCLES

To use strain-counterstrain techniques on these muscles, lie on your side with your head on a low pillow. These points lie at the base of your skull, in a hollow just to the side of the centre of the back of the neck (see Figure 9.1).

- Palpate the tender point on the side resting on the pillow using the hand on that same side, and press just hard enough to register the pain and score this in your mind as a '10'.
- The muscles at the base of the skull, when tender, need for the head to be taken backwards and usually leaned, and perhaps turned, away from the side of pain to ease the tenderness you are causing by your pressure.
- First, just take the head *slightly* backwards, very slowly, as though you are looking upwards. If the palpated pain changes, give it a score. If it is now *below* '10', you are working along the right lines. Bend your neck backwards

**Figure 9.1** *Palpating the tender point in the suboccipital muscles (where Rectus capitis posterior minor muscle is situated) – see Chapter 4.*

a little further, very slowly, and then allow the head to
tum and perhaps lean a little way away from the painful
side. Keep fine-tuning the position in this way and
you should slowly reduce the pain score. You should
eventually find a position in which it is reduced to 3 or
less. If you follow these directions and do not achieve
such a score reduction, the particular dynamics of your
muscular pain might need you to turn the head towards
the side where you feel pain or to find some other slight
variation of position to achieve ease.

- Once you have found the position of maximum ease, just
  relax in that position. Also, at this point you do not need
  to maintain pressure on the tender point all the time,
  just test it from time to time by pressing, to make sure it
  is still easy, that is, less painful.

- Remember also that the position which eases the
  tenderness should not produce any other pain – you
  should be relatively comfortable when resting with the
  pain point at ease.

- Stay like this for at least one minute and then *slowly*
  return to a neutral position, tum over and treat the
  other side in the same way.

## THE SIDE OF THE NECK

The points in this region lie near the side of the base of the neck
between the fifth and seventh cervical vertebrae (see Figure 9.2
on page 218).

- You can find the location of the tenderness by running
  a finger very lightly – just skin on skin, no pressure –
  down the side of your neck, starting just below the ear
  lobe. As you run down, you should be able to feel the
  slight 'bump' as you pass over the tips of the transverse
  processes of the vertebrae, that is, the part of the

**Figure 9.2** *Palpating for tender points in the muscles attaching to the transverse processes of the neck.*

vertebrae that sticks out sideways. When you get to the level of your neck which is about level with your chin, start to press in lightly after each 'bump' trying to find an area of tenderness on one side of your neck.

- Once you have found this, sit or lie down and allow the head to bend forwards (use a cushion to support your head if you are lying on your back).

- You should find that tenderness will be reduced as you take the head forwards. Find the most 'easy' position by experimenting with different amounts of forward bending.

- The tenderness will be reduced even more as you fine-tune the position of your head and neck by bending sideways slightly and turning the head either towards or away from the side where the pain is – whichever gives the best results in terms of your 'pain score'.

- When you get the score down to a 3 or less, stay in that position for at least a minute and then slowly return to a neutral position. Then, seek out a tender point on the outer side of the neck and treat it also.

## THE MIDPOINT OF THE UPPER TRAPEZIUS MUSCLE

The trapezius muscle runs from the neck to the shoulder.

- You can get easy access to tender points in this muscle by using a slight 'pinching' grip on the muscle, using your thumb and index finger of, say, the right hand to gently squeeze the muscle fibres between the base of the neck and the left shoulder until something very tender is found (see Figure 9.3).
- If pressure is maintained on this tender point for 3 or 4 seconds, it might well start to produce a radiating pain in a distant site, probably the head, in which case the *tender* point is also a *trigger* point (the same could be true of any of the tender points you are going to palpate,

**Figure 9.3** *Palpating (by squeezing) tender points lying in the upper trapezius muscle.*

but this position is one of the likeliest and commonest for which this is true).

- Lie down on the side that is the opposite to the one you are treating.
- Lightly pinch the point to produce a score of 10 and try altering the position of the arm, perhaps taking it up and over your head to 'slacken' the muscle you are palpating, or altering the neck position by having it bent sideways towards the painful side on a thick cushion. Fine-tune the arm and head positions until you reduce the score in your pain point (don't pinch it all the time, just intermittently to test whether a new position is allowing it to ease).
- Once you find your position of ease (with a score down to 3 or less), stay in that position for not less than a minute.
- Slowly return to a neutral position, sit up and seek out a tender point in the corresponding position on the other side of the body.

### WHERE THE SUPRASPINATUS MUSCLE ABOVE THE SHOULDER-BLADE BEGINS

The supraspinatus muscle lies along the top edge of the shoulder-blade.

- To find this muscle, lie on your back with your head flat on the floor or bed and, resting your elbow on your chest, ease your hand over your opposite shoulder area to feel with the tips of your fingers for the upper surface (nearest your neck) of the shoulder-blade (see Figure 9.4).
- To find the tender point, run your fingers along this upper surface towards the spine until you come to the end of the shoulder-blade and there, press into the muscles a little, looking for an area of great tenderness (most of us are tender here). You may need to press a little down or back towards the shoulder or in some

**Figure 9.4** *Palpating for tender points in supraspinatus muscle near the upper surface of the shoulder-blade.*

other direction until you find what you are looking for and can score the sensitivity as a '10'.

■ With the arm of the affected side resting at your side and while your finger remains in contact with the tender point, bend the arm on the affected side so that your fingertips rest close to your shoulder.

■ Now bring the elbow on the affected side up towards the ceiling, very slowly, and let it fall slightly away from the shoulder, about half-way down towards the surface on which you are lying. Does this reduce the score?

■ It should. Now start to fine-tune the arm position by rotating the bent arm gently at the shoulder, twisting so that the elbow comes towards the chest and the hand moves away from the shoulder, ever so slightly, until the pain is down to a score of about 3. Hold this position for at least a minute, then slowly return to a neutral position before doing the same on the other side of your body.

■ Sitting in a chair, rest your middle finger on the upper border of your breastbone and move it slowly sideways until you touch the end of your collar-bone where it joins your breastbone. Now run the finger along your collar-bone towards your shoulder for not more than 2.5 cm (1 in), and then down towards the chest 13 mm (½ in) or so and you should feel first a slight 'valley' and then you will come to the second rib (you cannot touch the first one because it is hidden behind the collar-bone). Press the upper surface of the second rib firmly and it should be tender, perhaps very tender (see Figure 9.5).

■ Maintain the pressure and score a '10' and then begin to take that score down by first bending the head and your upper back forwards, slightly (very slightly) towards the side of the pain point, until you feel the pain reduce.

■ Find the most 'easy' position of this forward movement, bending slightly to the side, and then see whether slightly tilting the head one way or the other helps to

**Figure 9.5** *Palpating for tender points in second intercostal muscles (between the ribs) close to where the rib meets the sternum (breastbone).*

reduce the score even more. Try also to take a full deep breath in, then slowly let the breath go and see which part of the breathing cycle eases the tenderness most.

- Once you have the score down to a 3 or less, add in the most 'easy' phase of the breath (hold the breath at that phase which eases the pain most) for 10 to 15 seconds. Then breathe normally, but maintain the position of ease for at least a minute before slowly returning to a neutral position and seeking out the tender point on the other side of the body to treat in the same way.

After trying this form of self-treatment out on these 10 points (5 on each side), you can now use the strain-counterstrain technique to treat any other painful point or muscle using these same methods. The relief experienced will be variable, lasting for a short or long period depending on what caused the pain. At least you have a practical first aid measure.

Remember the basic rules:

- find a pain point score 10
- move the body or part of the body around slowly until the pain has reduced to a 3
- hold for a minute
- slowly return to a neutral position.

That's all there is to strain-counterstrain, and it works.

By also using the muscle energy technique described in the previous chapter, you have the means with which to release tense, tight, stiff and restricted muscles without there being any danger.

## Myofascial release techniques
A range of manual methods known as myofascial release techniques have been suggested as being useful in treatment and rehabilitation of FMS.

In their book *Myofascial Manipulation*, physical therapists Robert Cantu and Alan Grodin state, 'Myofascial manipulation is one of the early aspects of therapeutic management of fibromyalgia . . . [which] should include appropriate elongation and stretching techniques. Joint restrictions should be addressed, concurrently with the soft tissue restrictions . . . Early in the program the clinician should instruct the patient in appropriate stretching exercises.' They go on to recommend Feldenkrais and Alexander techniques and state that, 'early cardiovascular [aerobic] training should be started' (R. Cantu and A. Grodin, 1992).

In general these recommendations are in line with the evidence from research, that gentle mobilization of stiff and restricted areas plus self stretching and exercise are usually helpful (see notes on aerobics in the next chapter).

# 10

# What Seems to Work in Treating Fibromyalgia?

Sidney Block, MD, a leading American rheumatologist, does not believe that fibromyalgia is a real condition that can be separated from what he calls 'generalized rheumatism', and he has argued this case in numerous articles (1993). As indicated in earlier chapters, this opinion is not universal and many people do see fibromyalgia as being a distinct condition, even if it blurs into chronic fatigue syndrome (ME) in many people's estimation.

Indeed, Robert Bennett, MD, a leading researcher into fibromyalgia, says, 'I am in disagreement with Dr. Block's construct of "generalized rheumatism"', a position he goes on to defend vigorously, showing that, in many ways, fibromyalgia is unique, involving microtrauma of the muscles (1993). His partial answer to the problem involves 'training', by which he means exercise.

Research by Dr. D. Felson and Dr. Don Goldenberg involving a three-year observation of the histories of 39 fibromyalgia sufferers showed that, over this period of time, 60 per cent of them complained of continuing symptoms despite taking medication virtually constantly to control them (1986). Remissions were rare and short-lived.

Dr. Block discusses the waxing and waning nature of the symptoms and reports that about 20 per cent of sufferers with 'generalized rheumatism' achieve remissions that can last for a long time. He believes that therapy should be aimed at alleviating the symptoms where possible and helping sufferers to cope better.

Others believe there is more on offer than this limited, if praiseworthy, set of objectives.

One of the problems Dr. Block raises relates to the evidence for the success or failure of different approaches. Most were found to have some value, but most also did not improve the lot of a large number of the fibromyalgia sufferers. He quotes from F. Wolf, whose research shows, for example, that in a selected group of sufferers, the results of treatment were as shown in Table 10.1 (1986) opposite.

This useful summary of information from 1986 gives us a lot to think about.

We can see that while *all* forms of treatment helped some sufferers, of those who tried rest, relaxation, physical treatment and chiropractic, more people benefited than did not benefit.

In the groups using the much-touted antidepressant medication, for example, there were more sufferers left feeling that they did *not* benefit than those that did. The same was found in the exercise group.

The results of the exercise and physical therapy are surprising, but as the forms of exercise and physical therapy used in the research were not specified, it is not possible to say why this was the case.

What we can conclude from this research is that *everything* helps *someone* and some methods help some people more than others.

In this chapter, some of the conventional and alternative methods commonly used to treat fibromyalgia will be examined and reported on. Although the variety of choices available may seem to lead to confusion, what emerges from this review is that both orthodox medical approaches to treatment and a host of alternative ones seem to offer hope and relief, if not an absolute guarantee of success for every sufferer.

**Table 10.1** F. Wolf's findings from research into the results of treatment received by fibromyalgia sufferers

| Treatment method | % of patients | % of those who tried this treatment method | |
|---|---|---|---|
| | | *no improvement* | *moderate to great improvement* |
| Exercise | 86.8 | 40.9 | 25.0 |
| Relaxation | 84.2 | 21.8 | 46.8 |
| Rest | 97.3 | 15.1 | 65.7 |
| Vacation | 76.3 | 53.4 | 29.3 |
| Painkilling drugs | 88.2 | 46.3 | 45.8 |
| Narcotics | 61.5 | 45.8 | 45.8 |
| Steroid injections | 52.6 | 45.0 | 36.0 |
| Tranquillizers | 28.6 | 28.6 | 23.8 |
| Antidepressants | 51.5 | 51.5 | 36.3 |
| Amitriptyline (bedtime low dose) | 51.0 | 56.6 | 30.2 |
| Physical therapy | 37.5 | 31.5 | 37.5 |
| Chiropractic | 48.7 | 16.2 | 45.9 |

If you are thinking why or how can so many different methods of treating the body possibly all be successful, return to the opening discussions in Chapters 6 and 7 (especially that relating to homeostasis). Essentially, it is because the only healing that ever takes place is that which the body's own repair and defence mechanisms produce and so 'treatment' (other than that aimed purely at symptom control) needs to be directed at removing obstacles to the recovery of health.

Which particular obstacles are being removed and/or which aspects of the homeostatic mechanisms are being enhanced will determine (and will be determined by) what form the treatment takes and whether the treatment is acting on a structural, functional, mechanical, biochemical, psychological, energetic or other level.

The variety of choices open to you for treatment relates to the many interacting causes involved in fibromyalgia and chronic fatigue syndrome (ME). Therefore, a degree of careful evaluation and selection is required before a course of treatment is decided on, and the decisions need to be based on the evidence available to date.

Some sufferers respond well to homoeopathic medication, others to herbal approaches.

Most will benefit (but to varying degrees) from appropriate body work (especially non-invasive osteopathic methods), chiropractic and acupuncture.

Many will benefit from a careful use of drugs that modify their sleep patterns.

Various other approaches have also claimed success in treating fibromyalgia and chronic fatigue syndrome (ME), ranging from healing (therapeutic touch or 'faith' healing) and hypnotherapy to biofeedback and forms of psychotherapy, such as cognitive-behavioural modification programmes.

The discussion of the available options in this chapter is not exhaustive – there are bound to be methods of treatment that are not covered here – but the breadth of what is included should allow for a considered and intelligent choice to be made when deciding what might be a desirable course of action, apart from the self-help measures and constitutional approaches covered in previous chapters.

*Caution:* Note that the inclusion of a particular method in this chapter should not be taken as being a recommendation for its use in your particular circumstances. This discussion is an exploration of what is being claimed in what appear to be responsible publications by a wide range of therapists and practitioners. However, there is no absolute 'quality control' and it is not possible to adequately compare the accuracy of the reports on which these discussions are based. Therefore, it is suggested that you make choices only after careful consideration and expert advice.

## Acupuncture

Acupuncture in general and electroacupuncture in particular have excellent track records in the treatment of pain (DeLuze, 1992, and Sandford Kiser, 1983). The basic techniques go back thousands of years, but the modem refinements, along with our increased understanding of how pain works and the various methods of modifying or obliterating it, all come together to make this a method that should be useful in the management of most muscular pain problems, including fibromyalgia.

One of the leading experts in the use of acupuncture in pain relief is Dr. P. Baldry and in his book *Acupuncture, Trigger Points and Musculosleketal Pain* (1993), he devotes some considerable space to consideration of fibromyalgia and myofascial pain syndrome. After asserting categorically that acupuncture is certainly the treatment of choice for dealing with myofascial pain syndrome or trigger point problems, he states:

> The pain in FMS – which would seem to be due to some as yet unidentified noxious substance in the circulation giving rise to neural hyperactivity at tender points and trigger points – takes a protracted course and it is only possible by means of acupuncture to suppress this neural hyperactivity for short periods.

He writes that it is necessary in treating fibromyalgia to repeat treatment every two to three weeks for months or even years, which he regards as being unsatisfactory, 'but nevertheless some patients insist that it improves the quality of their lives'.

Relief from pain for weeks on end and an enhanced quality of life would seem quite desirable objectives and results, perhaps helping ease the pain burden while more fundamental approaches are dealing with constitutional and causative issues.

A Swiss research team in Geneva has examined the effectiveness of electroacupuncture in treating fibromyalgia (DeLuze, *et al.*, 1992). A group of 70 sufferers (54 women) who all met the American College of Rheumatology criteria for fibromyalgia received either sham acupuncture ('wrong' points used) or the real thing. Various methods were used for patients to record their level of symptom activity and the amount of medication they used before and after treatment. Their sleep quality, morning stiffness and pain were all monitored.

Over a three-week period, the electroacupuncture treatment was administered with only the doctor giving the treatment knowing whether or not the needles were being placed correctly and whether or not the amount and type of electrical current being passed through the needles was correct.

Seven out of the eight measurements showed that only the group receiving real acupuncture felt notable benefits from the treatment. As in all such studies, a few minor improvements are always noted in the dummy or placebo group, but these were only slight in this study.

After treatment, the group receiving real acupuncture required far more pressure on tender points to produce pain and the amount of painkilling medication they needed was virtually halved, as were their assessments of regional pain levels. There was also a significant increase in their quality of sleep. The length of time morning stiffness was experienced only reduced by a small amount.

Around 25 per cent of the group receiving the real treatment did not improve significantly, but all the others showed remarkable levels of improvement, with some experiencing almost complete relief from all their symptoms. The duration of the improvement was 'several weeks' in most patients, which seems to be in line with Dr. Baldry's observation of it being necessary to repeat treatment every few weeks.

The fact that there are virtually no side-effects from electroacupuncture makes it attractive when compared with painkilling and/or antidepressant medication.

In more recent research at UCLA it has been found that injecting active trigger points with the pain-killing agent xylocaine produced marked benefits in FMS patients in terms of pain relief and reduction of stiffness, but that this is not really significantly apparent for at least a week after the injections. FMS patients reported more local soreness following the injections than patients with only myofascial pain (see discussion in Chapter 4 regarding the role of trigger points in FMS), but improved after this settled down. This reinforces the opinion of many practitioners that myofascial trigger points contribute a large degree of the pain being experienced in FMS (C. Hong, 1996).

### Aerobic exercise

Cardiovascular exercise, as we have seen, is reported to be helpful as a means of recovery from fibromyalgia.

The guidelines most commonly given to sufferers to ensure that it will have a beneficial effect is that aerobic exercise be performed 3 times weekly (some say 4 times) for at least 20 (some say 15) minutes each session, during which time you need to achieve between 60 and 85 per cent of your maximum predicted heart rate.

The forms of aerobic exercise best suited to fibromyalgia sufferers are said to be cycling (using an exercise bike), walking or swimming. Appropriate warm-up and cool-down periods are suggested, and a slow, incremental programme is needed to reach the prescribed length and frequency of exercising.

Exercising encourages the body to release its own pain-killing hormone-like substances (endorphins) and so exercising can bring about some pain relief and enhance well-being, increase self-esteem and give a psychological boost as fitness increases.

A study involving 34 fibromyalgia sufferers had some of the patients perform aerobic exercise (cycling, designed to achieve a heart rate of 150 per minute) or flexibility exercises (achieving no more than 115 beats per minute) 3 times a week for 20 weeks (McCain, 1986). At the end of this period, those doing the aerobic routines achieved a far greater reduction in pain than did those doing the flexibility exercises.

A Swedish study compared groups of FMS patients who over a six-week period were given (six one-hour) educational lectures about their condition and how to manage it, with a group who attended these same lectures but who also received (six one-hour) sessions of physical training (C. Burckhardt *et al.*, 1994). A further group (used to compare the effect of doing something with doing nothing in similar patients) were untreated during this entire study but received treatment after it was over. The results (86 patients completed the study) showed that both the lecture and the lecture plus exercise groups showed a positive impact on their quality of life as well as their pain levels. However, it was those who performed the active exercises who were shown to maintain the benefits long term more effectively. Eighty-seven per cent reported that they were exercising at least three times weekly for 20 minutes or more. Around 70 per cent were practising relaxation techniques. A number had been able to return to work as a result of the programme.

In another study, the benefits of exercise (fitness, flexibility and strengthening) programmes were compared with relaxation exercises in a group of 60 FMS patients over a six-week period at the Medical School of the University of Calgary, Canada. Both groups of patients (those doing active exercise, and those doing relaxation) met three times a week for six weeks to carry out their routines under supervision. At the start both groups had the same amount of pain, stiffness, etc. Of the 30 people starting the exercises, 18 completed the course along with 20 (of the 30) in the relaxation group. Both groups showed an improvement in the number and sensitivity of tender points, but those doing the active training exercises were much improved compared with the relaxation group.

What this study shows is that a number of people (around a third) fall out of such programmes for one reason or another. Those that complete their assignments usually benefit, and exercising appropriately is very beneficial in FMS (Martin *et al.*, 1996).

See Chapter 8 once more for the discussion regarding the possibility that some people with chronic fatigue syndrome (ME) are unable to do any exercise at all in some stages of their illness.

See also Cognitive-behavioural treatment below. In this form of treatment, tasks and routines (which have been agreed and negotiated between the chronic fatigue sufferer and the therapist) are performed daily with slight increments over time, however the person feels (on good days and bad days), but always staying just inside what is possible without strain.

## Chiropractic

There is a mass of anecdotal reporting of the benefit of chiropractic treatment of fibromyalgia and chronic fatigue syndrome (ME). Few clinical studies support these claims, but, as the manipulative methodologies of osteopathy and chiropractic have become ever closer and as the methods of osteopathy that focus on muscles – notably strain-counterstrain and muscle energy treatment – are now widely used by massage therapists and as there are clinical studies of osteopathic manipulative therapy and massage (see below), it is safe to assume that the anecdotal claims are accurate.

Those forms of chiropractic that focus on muscles – such as Morter's bio-energetic synchronization technique (BEST) – are more likely to be helpful in fibromyalgia than the more active adjustment methods. These latter techniques, though, do have their place when joint restrictions are a prominent symptom.

Recent research at Canadian Memorial Chiropractic College, in Toronto, involved 21 fibromyalgia patients who received four weeks of chiropractic manipulation, soft tissue treatment and stretching, based on the individual needs as assessed by the chiropractor. During the first four weeks half the patients received treatment, and during the second four weeks the other half of the group received chiropractic treatment. This was done to evaluate the benefits of active as against no treatment (apart from whatever medication was being taken, which continued throughout whether chiropractic treatment was being received or not). The outcome was that there were definite improvements in those receiving chiropractic in terms of increased mobility and pain reduction. It is obviously not possible to say which aspects of the treatment were helpful, since soft tissue and joint manipulation were both applied (K. Blunt, 1997).

## Cognitive-behavioural treatment

It is generally agreed that the differences between fibromyalgia and chronic fatigue syndrome (ME) are marginal at best and that many – probably most – patients in each category could just as easily be diagnosed as having one of the other conditions.

One model of these conditions suggests that whatever the trigger (trauma, viral infection, toxicity and so on), there needs also to be perpetuating factors, such as emotional stress, inadequate rest patterns or concurrent depression, say. This treatment approach suggests tackling the behavioural and cognitive aspects, using agreed targets (agreed between therapist and sufferer) for changing the behaviour pattern that has become established by the illness (Beck, 1979, Deale and Wessley, 1994).

Careful planning and preparation are required, with a lot of attention being paid to engaging the sufferer in the process of their own recovery. The sufferer is not led to believe that this is *all* there is to treatment, but is encouraged to see that while underlying factors (a virus or whatever) are being dealt with, the perpetuating factors can begin to be modified. A gradual increase in activity is the aim, with an equally gradual reduction in rest periods. The key to success is not to do too much too soon, staying within what is a manageable level for the sufferer. A structured schedule evolves via negotiation and discussion over 20 to 30 sessions. The same degree of activity is suggested on good and bad days, with perhaps no increase in activity initially, but a structured pattern emerging. Very gradually, activity increases and responsibility for what happens is transferred fully to the patient.

Does it work? Some claim it does, but it takes dedication on every one's part.

### Combined (group) treatment

Research at the Department of Medicine, Oregon Health Sciences University in the USA evaluated the impact of six months (one hour per week) of group treatment involving lectures and group sessions of active fitness training, stress reduction, relaxation, behaviour modification and flexibility (stretching exercises) (R. Bennett *et al.*, 1996). A questionnaire was used to evaluate the impact of FMS on the person's life; their total tender point score was also measured regularly. Also measured were levels of fitness (how far could they walk in six minutes?), depression scores, quality of life scores, etc. Between 15 and 25 patients turned up regularly and their condition was monitored for two years after the end of the six months of the trial. Over a four-year period, 170 patients took part in the study, with 104 completing the full six months during their time on the programme.

The findings were:

■ After six months on this combined group programme 70 per cent of those completing it had reduced their number of tender points to less than 11.

- There was a 25 per cent improvement in the impact of fibromyalgia on their lives.
- After two years, 33 patients who were questioned and examined showed continued improvement.
- Approximately 30 people who never entered the programme were followed to have something to compare those in the active group with. These non-active FMS patients showed no improvement over the same period.

### Dry needling and injection into trigger points

There have been few clinical trials of bodywork treatment of fibromyalgia. However, there is abundant evidence of the successful use of various methods for treating trigger points, including the injection of saline or Procaine or even simply 'dry needling' (for example using a hypodermic needle without injecting anything, like acupuncture with normal needles) the trigger points. In one study, 46 per cent of those people with fibromyalgia given this latter form of treatment found that this approach offered them the longest lasting relief of symptoms compared with other forms of treatment they had received. Also, 69 per cent of them required less medication for some time afterwards.

### Herbal medicine

There have been no clinical trials of herbal treatment of fibromyalgia, but, as mentioned in Chapter 6, at least one very well-researched herb is being used clinically to help circulation to the brain – *Ginkgo biloba* (more on this herb below).

In addition, leading herbalists are on record as claiming benefits from an approach that tries to 'support the nervous system with herbal nerve tonics and adaptogens' (the latter are substances that help the body cope with stress). Additionally, herbal methods try to help the defence mechanisms by using known immune system enhancers, such as echinacea, astragalus and ginseng.

Various nervine herbs would also be included in a combination aimed at helping normalize sleep.

A valuable herbal combination formula is (Kacera, 1993):

2 parts *Panax quinquefolium* (American ginseng)
2 parts *Astragalus mongolicus*
2 parts *Angelica sinensis* (dong quai)
1 part *Ginkgo biloba*
1 part *Cimicfuga racemosa* (black cohosh)
½ part *Passiflora incarnata* (passion flower)
½ part *Betonica officinalis* (wood betony)
½ part *Matricaria chamomila* (chamomile)
½ part *Zizyphus sativa* (jujube red dates).

This formulation is claimed to be a tonic that will support people with chronic weakness, anxiety, headaches, sleep disturbances and general fatigue, as well as diminished blood flow to the extremities. The person who needs this will probably have a weak pulse, weak digestive system, headaches and be fatigued.

A dose of between half and one teaspoon, two or three times daily, taken between meals is suggested.

*Gingko biloba* is a herb (just the leaves are used, not the fruit) that deserves more attention and the following information may encourage its wider use in the treatment of fibromyalgia and chronic fatigue syndrome (ME). The benefits may take some months to be noticed in chronic cases, but among the scientifically proven effects of this herb are:

- improved short-term memory
- enhanced cerebral blood flow
- reduction in vertigo
- reduction in ischemia (poor oxygenation of tissues)
- reduction in oxidative processes (it acts as an antioxidant)
- antibacterial activity.

A large group of people with memory loss were treated with this herb in a London hospital and given doses of 120 mg daily, a third of this being taken three times a day, and their ability to remember things improved (Kleijnen, 1992).

In other trials as much as 600 mg was given daily. There were no side-effects and memory enhancement and improved reaction times were observed, indicating improved functioning of the brain, probably because of better circulation (Warot, 1991).

### Homoeopathy

Several studies have looked at the effects of a specific homoeopathic remedy, Rhus tox, in treating fibromyalgia and 'fibrositis' and the results have been variable.

It is necessary to understand the basis of homoeopathic prescribing in order to make sense of the different results in the trials of this substance, so here, very briefly, are the principles.

Homoeopathic remedies comprise minute quantities of substances that in larger amounts would produce very similar or identical symptoms to those being experienced. The substance is then used in an extremely diluted form to treat the symptoms of the condition in people whose temperament and personality, as well as numerous other characteristics, fit the picture of the people most affected by the medication in past trials.

When a remedy is selected in classical homoeopathy, therefore, it is not just the *symptoms* that are taken into account but a 'constitutional profile' of the person affected, that is, their whole state of 'health'. This means that while two people might have the same named condition – say asthma – they might require *different* remedies if they have different personalities, likes and dislikes, and were affected differently by particular factors. Thus, although treatment of painful rheumatic conditions by homoeopathy often involves the use of Rhus tox, it is not suitable for *all* people with such conditions, only those with the profile that matches the medicine.

So, the ideal person to take Rhus tox has the following characteristics:

- restless, continually changing position, apprehensive, especially at night, and finds it difficult to stay in bed
- the head will feel heavy, and the jaws may be noisy, creaking, with pain in the tempero-mandibular joint
- the tongue tends to be coated, except for a red triangular area near the tip, and there is a frequently bitter taste in the mouth and a desire for milky drinks
- there is often a drowsy feeling after eating
- there may be a nagging, dry cough and a sense of palpitation that is most noticeable when sitting still
- the back tends to be stiff and normally feels better for moving about
- the limbs are stiff and any exposure to cold makes the skin feel sensitive or painful
- cold, wet weather makes the symptoms worse, as does sleep and resting
- what helps most as far as symptoms are concerned is warm, dry weather, movement, rubbing the uncomfortable areas, warm applications and stretching.

For this profile, the remedy is Rhus tox 6C potency, but *only* for this profile!

## THE TRIALS OF RHUS TOX

In Britain, a study found that using the 6C dilution of Rhus tox was effective in moderating the symptoms of patients with fibromyalgia, but a trial in Australia, involving just three patients who fitted all the criteria, including the profile for Rhus tox, found that there was no benefit when a 6X dilution was used (Fisher, 1989, and Gemmell, 1991). The difference between 6X and 6C dilutions may seem unimportant, but it is actually enormous.

To make a 1C dilution, 1 part of the substance is vigorously mixed with 99 parts of ethanol (an alcohol used to preserve the substance). To make a 2C dilution, 1 drop of the first mix is placed with another 99 drops of ethanol and the process is repeated. By the time you get to 6C, the dilution is minute, and this is what was used in the first study mentioned. Paradoxically this is called a high potency and is considered more powerful and faster acting in terms of triggering a healing response than a low potency.

'X' potencies are low – only 1 drop of the substance to 9 drops of ethanol are needed to make 1X, with the process being repeated 5 more times to make 6X, which was used in the second trial mentioned above.

With one study using Rhus tox 6C and claiming marked benefits for fibromyalgia sufferers and one using Rhus tox 6X showing no benefit, the jury is still out. However, as there is absolutely no chance of side effects with homoeopathy, there is little to be lost in trying – but try the 6C dilution if you have the above profile and want to give it a try.

### Hypnotherapy

In controlled trials, it has been found that hypnotherapy helps more than physical therapy in those sufferers who do not seem to respond well to most other forms of treatment. Pain is reduced, fatigue and stiffness on waking are improved and their general feeling of well-being is better (Haanen, 1991).

### Massage

Research at the Touch Research Institute, Miami School of Medicine, in 1994 has shown that fibromyalgia responds well to massage (*Touch Therapy Times*, 1994). There they took 30 adults diagnosed with the condition and divided them into three groups. The first group received massage for 30 minutes twice a week for 5 weeks. The second group received TENS treatment (this is when electrical impulses are applied to a painful area to mask the pain), also for

30 minutes twice a week for 5 weeks. The third group received dummy TENS treatment the same number of times and over the same period of time as the second group.

Rheumatologists evaluated the results by assessing the changes that occurred in the sufferers' tender points and found that all groups showed some reduction in the number of points that were painful, but only those receiving massage reported decreases in pain, fatigue, stiffness and improvements in the quality of sleep.

## VIBRATIONAL MASSAGE

Massage researcher Richard Van Why (1994) reports that studies at Sweden's Karolinska Institute have shown that mechanical vibration applied to a pain point for 15 to 30 minutes (at 100 to 200 cycles per second) will powerfully relieve pain and cause the release of long-held tensions in the muscles. Using the hands to vibrate the skin, by using firm pressure plus a rapid vibration, appears to produce the same bene fits without causing any negative effects.

## Medication

The most widespread treatment given for fibromyalgia involves the use of various pharmacological agents and it is useful to evaluate the results of studies as to their efficacy.

Tricyclic antidepressant medications increase the amount of serotonin in the central nervous system, increase the delta-wave stage of sleep and consistently improve the symptoms of fibromyalgia, though not by acting as an antidepressant and not in all sufferers treated.

Studies involving various forms of antidepressant medication tend to support the use of amitriptyline (25 to 50 mg daily), with pain scores, stiff ness, sleep and fatigue symptoms all improving on average, but by no means in all sufferers (Carette, 1986).

In one study, 77 per cent of fibromyalgia sufferers receiving amitriptyline reported general improvement after 5 weeks. Only

43 per cent of those receiving placebo medication could say the same (Goldenberg, 1986).

Side-effects of taking the antidepressant were measurable, however, with drowsiness, confusion, seizure, agitation, nightmares, blurred vision, hallucinations, uneven heartbeat, gastrointestinal upsets, low blood pressure, constipation, urinary retention, impotence and dryness of the mouth all being observed or reported in various combinations.

When combined with osteopathic manipulative methods (see below), antidepressant medication offers greater relief.

A study of the use of systemic corticosteroids (15 mg daily of prednisone) showed that there were no measurable improvements in those taking them and, as side-effects are usual with such medication, this form of treatment is clearly not desirable (Clark, 1985). Indeed, if it were to produce an improvement it would still be sensible to question whether fibromyalgia was indeed the correct diagnosis as the symptoms of some other rheumatic condition are more likely to improve with its use.

When muscle relaxants were tested as treatment for fibromyalgia sufferers, most were found to be useless. However, cyclobenzaprine (10 to 40 mg daily, given at night to prevent daytime drowsiness) was found to reduce pain levels and tender point count and improve sleep (Campbell, 1985). It is thought that it has this effect because it has a chemical similarity to amitriptyline.

Many other drugs are being researched and tried as treatments for fibromyalgia, ranging from antiviral agents to substances that modulate the immune system. Various cocktails of antidepressant and sedative medications are being tried out as well. Even aspirin has been tried and is said to be mildly useful.

### Osteopathy
Practitioners of osteopathic treatment, from which both strain-counterstrain and muscle energy treatment derive (see Chapters

8 and 9), have conducted many studies into fibromyalgia. Among the most recent are the following.

Doctors at Chicago College of Osteopathic Medicine, led by Drs A. Stotz and R. Keppler, measured the effects of osteopathic manipulative therapy (OMT, which includes strain-counterstrain and muscle energy treatment) on the intensity of pain from tender points in 18 people who met all the criteria for fibromyalgia (Stotz, 1993).

Each had 6 treatments and it was found that, over a year, 12 of them responded well in that their tender points became less sensitive (a 14 per cent reduction against a 34 per cent increase in the 6 patients who did not respond well).

Most of the sufferers – the responders and the non-responders to OMT – showed that their tender points were more symmetrically spread after the course (their positions being established using thermographic imaging) than before. Their ability to perform the activities of daily living were significantly improved and general pain symptoms decreased.

Doctors at Texas College of Osteopathic Medicine selected three groups of fibromyalgia sufferers, one of which received OMT, another had OMT plus self-teaching (study of the condition and self-help measures) and a third group received only moist heat treatment (Jiminez, 1993). The group with the least reported pain after six months of care was that receiving OMT – although benefits were also noted in the self-teaching group.

Another group of doctors from Texas tested the difference in results of 3 types of treatment as given to 37 fibromyalgia sufferers (Rubin, *et al.*, 1990). The methods were drugs only (ibuprofen, alprazolam) or OMT plus medication or a dummy medication (placebo) plus OMT or a placebo only.

The results showed that drug therapy alone resulted in significantly less tenderness being reported than did drugs and manipulation or the use of a placebo and OMT or placebo alone.

However, sufferers receiving a placebo plus manipulation reported significantly less fatigue than those in the other groups, and those receiving medication and OMT showed the greatest improvement in their quality of life.

At Kirksville, Missouri College of Osteopathic Medicine, 19 people meeting all the criteria of fibromyalgia were treated once a week for 4 weeks using OMT (Rubin, *et al.*, 1990). After this time, 84.2 per cent showed improved sleep patterns, 94.7 per cent reported less pain and most patients had fewer tender points on palpation.

Claims are made for the value of cranial osteopathic treatment, but there are no trials on which to base a value judgement, only anecdotal reports from satisfied patients.

## Supplementation

People with fibromyalgia and chronic fatigue syndrome (ME) are often found to be deficient in magnesium. In a study, 15 fibromyalgia sufferers were given 300 to 600 mg of magnesium supplements daily, plus 1200 to 1400 mg per day of malic acid (Abraham, 1992). Pain levels were greatly reduced, but it took some weeks or even months before such benefits were felt.

This study replicates a previous study that showed that magnesium deficiency was a feature of many patients with chronic fatigue syndrome (ME).

Research studies which show benefit of supplementation in chronic muscle pain conditions in general and fibromyalgia in particular include:

- 81 patients who were disabled with chronic stiffness, muscular pain and aching were treated with 140 micrograms of selenium and 100 mg of vitamin E daily, or dummy tablets (placebo).
- Pain relief was significantly greater in the muscle pain patients. These nutrients are antioxidants (as are vitamins A and C) which reduce damaging oxidation

processes which occur in many inflammatory and painful conditions (S. Jameson *et al.*, 1985).

- In Sweden, 44 patients with a diagnosis of FMS were prescribed 800 mg of S-adenosyl-L-methionine (SAMe) daily for six weeks, or a placebo. The symptoms which improved in those receiving SAMe as compared with the placebo were fatigue, morning stiffness, pain (not until the sixth week of treatment) and feelings of well-being (S. Jacobsen *et al.*, 1991).

- A review of current literature has shown that research is indicating high levels of an amino acid, homocysteine, in the cerebro-spinal fluid of people with fibromyalgia and CFS. There is an intimate relationship between homocysteine and SAMe as well as vitamins $B_6$ and $B_{12}$. This same review also indicates lower levels than normal of vitamin $B_{12}$ in the cerebro-spinal fluid of fibromyalgia patients – suggesting that SAMe supplementation along with $B_{12}$ might be a useful strategy – confirmed by the research summarized above (G. Kwiat, 1998).

- 50 patients with primary fibromyalgia syndrome were supplemented with either 5-hydroxytryptophan (100 mg three times daily) or a placebo for 30 days. After 30 days all the signs and symptoms in the treated group (compared with the placebo group) had improved significantly (fewer tender points, less pain, less stiffness, improved sleep, less anxiety and more energy) (I. Caruso *et al.*, 1990).

Additional supplementation strategies that are recommended as a result of clinical study include vitamins $B_3$ and $B_6$, which, together with magnesium and tryptophan (obtainable from a good protein meal), are needed to manufacture serotonin. Ornithine and arginine (see Chapter 6) can be used to promote growth hormone production.

Taking calcium and zinc supplements is commonly found to help sleep patterns return to normal.

Supplements that help support your general nutritional status include B complex and vitamin C, as well as essential fatty acids, derived from flax seeds or evening primrose.

Melatonin (3 mg) supplementation helps sleep patterns (and therefore growth hormone production). It is a mild natural antidepressant as well.

# 11

# Summary and Suggestions

The first and most vital aspect of all is to *get the right diagnosis*. You have to make sure that what you have is fibromyalgia and not one of the many other rheumatic-type problems, which can produce widespread muscular pain, such as polymyalgia rheumatica. Laboratory and other medical tests can identify most conditions that are *not* fibromyalgia.

Have expert advice as to how much of the problem might be related to trigger point activity, and whether or not myofascial pain syndrome is involved, as the pain from trigger points is relatively easy to eliminate using methods chosen from injections, acupuncture, bodywork and postural and/or breathing re-education.

Look at the various associated conditions and, using the advice given in Chapters 2 and 6 as a guide, try to have as many of these controlled or eliminated as possible – whether they be allergies, anxiety, hyperventilation, yeast or viral activity, bowel dysfunction, underactive thyroid, sleep disturbance or other conditions that are involved. Get expert advice from practitioners or therapists working with fibromyalgia sufferers.

As soon as possible, introduce as many of the constitutional health enhancement methods as you can – pranayama breathing followed by deep relaxation every day (autogenic training, for example), regular (weekly or fortnightly) detoxification days (which also boost growth hormone production), as described in Chapter 6, hydrotherapy (neutral bath whenever anxiety is a factor, and progressive cold bathing daily if fatigue or chronic pain are factors), regular, non-specific massage, if possible, and acupuncture for 'energy balancing', if available.

Get nutritional advice and improve your diet, as well as supplementing it if necessary. Use the nutritional pain relief measures described in Chapter 6, as well as general supplementation if there is any hint of deficiency, and consider the amino acid supplement methods for stimulating growth hormone production (see Chapter 6).

Consider introducing specific herbal help for circulation to the brain by taking *Ginkgo biloba* tablets regularly (available from any healthfood store) and perhaps taking homoeopathic Rhus tox 6C as well.

Get advice and treatment from an osteopath, chiropractor, physical therapist or licensed massage therapist regarding treatment of your muscular condition, and introduce regular (daily if possible) gentle self-treatment using strain-counterstrain and muscle energy treatment methods as described in Chapters 8 and 9.

Introduce regular exercise within your tolerance (take advice) and, if possible, include cardiovascular training and stretching movements (yoga and/or T'ai chi, say).

Use medication under medical advice only. Antidepressants are the most likely to give some benefit if taken in low dosages.

Join a support group, read all you can about your condition and health enhancement and start to take control of your condition, even if the progress is apparently slow. The more you understand the processes involved the better.

Consider your choices as to alternative and standard treatment methods, noting that, of all the methods, osteopathic bodywork, rest, exercise and mild medication along with acupuncture have the best track record.

Consider stress or general counselling in order to learn coping skills and stress-reduction tactics.

Be persistent and dedicated and, above all, live life at the pace currently available to you, but, within that framework, introduce set patterns of slowly increasing activity, even if fatigue is a major factor. You may have to negotiate this with yourself, setting simple, achievable targets and ensuring they are met, never involving excessive demands based on your current abilities. By slowly stretching your capabilities, you will regain both a greater range of potentials as well as confidence as you get better.

# Bibliography

Aarflot, T., 'Association between chronic widespread musculo-skeletal complaints and thyroid autoimmunity (community survey involving 1,500 individuals)', *Scandinavian Jnl Primary Health Care*, Vol. 14, No. 2, pp. 111–15, 1996.

Abraham, G., *et al.*, 'Management of FMS – rationale for the use of magnesium and malic acid', *Journal of Nutritional Medicine*, Vol. 3, pp. 49–59, 1992.

Affaitati, G., *et al.*, 'Effects of treatment of peripheral pain generators in fibromyalgia patients', *European Journal of Pain*, vol. 15 no. 1, pp. 61–69, 2011.

Amir, M., 'PTSD tenderness and fibromyalgia', *Journal of Psychosomatic Research*, Vol. 42, No. 6, pp. 607–13, 1997.

Balch, J., *Prescription for Nutritional Healing*, Avery, New York, 1990.

Baldry, P.E., *Acupuncture, Trigger Points and Musculoskeletal Pain*, Churchill Livingstone, London, 1993.

Beck, A., *et al.*, *Cognitive Therapy in Depression*, Guildford Press, New York, 1979.

Behan, P., 'Enteroviruses and post viral fatigue syndrome', in Bock, G. and Whelan, J. (eds), CFS CIBA Foundation Symposium 173, Wiley, 1993.

Bennett, Roger, 'Fibromyalgia: the facts', *Controversies in Clinical Rheumatism*, Vol. 19, No. 1, pp. 45–58, February 1993.

Bennett, R., *et al.*, 'Group treatment of FMS – a 6-month out-patient program', *Journal of Rheumatology*, Vol. 23, No. 3, pp. 521–8, 1996.

*Biomedical and Clinical Aspects of CoQ10*, Vol. 2, Elsevier Science, Amsterdam, 1980.

Bland, J., 'A medical food-supplemented detoxification programme in the management of chronic health problems', *Alternative Therapies*, Vol. 1, pp. 62–71, 1995.

Block, Sydney, 'Fibromyalgia and the rheumatisms', *Controversies in Clinical Rheumatology*, Vol. 19, No. 1, pp. 61–78, February, 1993.

Blunt, K., 'Effectiveness of chiropractic management of FMS – pilot study', *Journal of Manipulative Physiological Therapeutics*, Vol. 20, No. 6, pp. 389–400, 1997.

Brodin, H., 'Inhibition-facilitation technique', *Manual Medicine*, Vol. 3, pp. 24–36, 1987.

Buchwald, D., 'Comparison of patients with CFS, FMS and MCS', *Archives of Internal Medicine*, Vol. 154, No. 18, pp. 2049–53, 1994.

Buchwald, D., *et al.*, 'A chronic illness characterized by fatigue, neurologic and immunologic disorders and active human herpes virus type 6 infection', *Annals of Internal Medicine*, Vol. 116, pp. 103–13, 1992.

Burckhardt, C., *et al.*, 'Randomized controlled clinical trial of education and physical training for women with fibromyalgia', *Journal of Rheumatology*, Vol. 21, No. 4, pp. 714–20, 1994.

Burton, A., 'Therapeutic fasting' in *Textbook of Natural Medicine*, Pizzorno, J., and Murray, M. (eds), Bastyr University, Seattle, 1989.

Buskila, D., 'FMS in HIV Infection', *Journal of Rheumatology*, Vol. 17, pp. 1202–6, 1990.

Buskila, D., Neumann, L., *et al.*, 'Increased rates of fibromyalgia following cervical spine injury', *Arthritis and Rheumatism*, Vol. 40, No. 3, pp. 446–52, 1997.

Cantu, Robert, and Grodin, Alan, *Myofascial Manipulation*, Aspen Publications, Gaithersberg, Maryland, 1992.

Campbell, S., *et al.*, 'A double blind study of cyclobenzaprine in patients with primary fibromyalgia', *Arthritis and Rheumatology*, Vol. 28, section 40, 1985.

Carette, S., *et al.*, 'Evaluation of amitriptyline in primary fibrositis', *Arthritis and Rheumatology*, Vol. 29, pp. 655–9, 1986.

Caruso, I., *et al.*, 'Double blind study of 5-hydroxytryptophan versus placebo in treatment of primary FMS', *Journal of International Medical Research*, Vol. 18, No. 3, pp. 201–9, 1990.

Chaitow, L. (Medical Editor), *Alternative Medicine, Future Medicine*, San Francisco, 1994.

Chaitow, L., *Candida Albicans*, Thorsons, London, 1991.

Chaitow, L., *Natural Life Extension*, Thorsons, London, 1992.

Chaitow, L., *Soft Tissue Manipulation*, Thorsons, London, 1989.

Chaitow, L., *Stress Protection Plan*, Thorsons, London, 1992.

Chaitow, L., *Water Therapy*, Thorsons, London, 1994.

Chaitow, L., and Trenev, N., *Probiotics*, Thorsons, London, 1990.

Clark, S., *et al.*, 'Double blind crossover trial of prednisone in treatment of fibrositis', *Journal of Rheumatology*, Vol. 12, No. 5, pp. 980–3, 1985.

Clauw, D., 'Fibromyalgia: More than just a musculoskeletal disease', *American Family Physician*, September 1, 1995.

Cleveland, C., *et al.*, 'Chronic rhinitis and underrecognised association with fibromyalgia', *Allergy Proceedings*, Vol. 13, No. 5, pp. 263–7, 1992.

Consensus Document on FMS: The Copenhagen Declaration, *The Lancet*, Vol. 340, September 12, 1992.

Davies, S., *Nutritional Medicine*, Pan, London, 1987.

Deale, A., and Wessley, S., 'A cognitive-behavioural approach to CFS', *The Therapist*, Vol. 2, No. 1, pp. 11–14, 1994.

DeLuze, C., *et al.*, 'Electroacupuncture in fibromyalgia', *British Medical Journal*, Vol. 305, pp. 1249–52, 21 November 1992.

Dowsett, E., 'M.E. – a persistent viral infection?', *Postgraduate Medical Journal*, Vol. 66, pp. 526–30, 1990.

Duna, George, and Wilke, William, 'Diagnosis, etiology and therapy of fibromyalgia', *Comprehensive Therapy*, Vol. 19, No. 2, pp. 60–3, 1993.

Ediger, Beth, *Coping with Fibromyalgia*, LRH Publications, Toronto, 1991.

Ekici G., *et al.*, 'Comparison of manual lymph drainage therapy &

connective tissue massage, in women with fibromyalgia: a randomized controlled trial', *Journal of Manipulative and Physiological Therapeutics*, Vol. 32, pp. 127–133, 2009.

*The European*, 22 and 29 April, 1993 (report on research by the Thrombosis Research Institute into the effects of hydrotherapy).

Felson, D., and Goldenberg, Don, 'The natural history of fibromyalgia', *Arthritis and Rheumatology*, Vol. 29, pp. 1522–6, 1986.

Ferraccioli, G., 'Neuroendocrinologic findings in primary FMS', *Journal of Rheumatology*, Vol. 17, pp. 869–73, 1990.

Fibromyalgia Network Newsletters, October 1990 to January 1992, Compendium 2, January 1993, May 1993, Compendium, October 1993, January 1994, July 1994.

Fibromyalgia Network Newsletter, May 1993 Compendium (report on first national seminar for patients, Columbus, Ohio, April 1990, Dr. Robert Bennett's presentation on muscle microtrauma, pp. 23–5).

Fibromyalgia Network Newsletter , October 1997, pp. 11–13. (Back issues are available from the Network – PO Box 31750, Tucson, Arizona 85761–1750.)

Fisher, P., *et al.*, 'Effect of homoeopathic treatment of fibrositis (primary fibromyalgia)', *British Medical Journal*, Vol. 32, pp. 365–6, 1989.

Foster, S., *Ginkgo Botanical*, series 304, Austin Texas American Botanical Council, 1991.

Gardier, A., *et al.*, 'Effects of a primary immune response to T-cell dependent antigen on serotonin metabolism in the frontal cortex', *Brain Research*, Vol. 645, pp. 150–6, 1992.

Ge, H-Y *et al.*, 'Predetermined sites of examination for tender points in fibromyalgia syndrome are frequently associated with myofascial trigger points', *Journal of Pain,* Vol. 7, no. 11, pp. 644–651, 2010.

Gemmell, H., *et al.*, 'Homoeopathic Rhus toxicodendron in treatment of fibromyalgia', *Chiropractic Journal of Australia*, Vol. 21, No. 1, pp. 2–6, March 1991.

Goldenberg, Don, 'Fibromyalgia, chronic fatigue syndrome and myofascial pain syndrome', *Current Opinion in Rheumatology*, Vol. 5, pp. 199–208, 1993.

Goldenberg, D., 'Fibromyalgia and chronic fatigue syndrome', *Journal of*

*Musculoskeletal Pain*, Vol. 2, No. 3, pp. 51–5, 1994.

Goldenberg, D., *et al.*, 'Randomized, controlled trial of amitriptyline anproxine in treatment of patients with fibromyalgia', *Arthritis and Rheumatology*, Vol. 29, pp. 1371–7, 1986.

Goldstein, Jay, *Chronic Fatigue Syndrome: The limbic hypothesis*, Haworth Medical Press, Binghampton, New York, 1993.

Goldstein, J., *Betrayal by the Brain: The neurological basis of CFS and FM S and related neural network disorders*, The Haworth Medical Press, New York, 1996.

Gow, J., 'Enteroviral sequences detected in muscles of patients with postviral fatigue syndrome', *British Medical Journal*, Vol. 302, pp. 692–6, 1991.

Haanen, H., *et al.*, 'Controlled trial of hypnotherapy in treatment of refractory fibromyalgia', *Journal of Rheumatology*, Vol. 18, pp. 72–5, 1991.

Hack, G., Koritzer, R., Robinson, W., Hallgren, R., Greenman, P., 'Anatomic relationship between rectus capitis posterior minor muscle and the dura mater', *Spine*, Vol. 120, No. 23, pp. 2484–6, December 1995.

Hallgren, R., Greenman, P., Rechtien, J., 'MRI of normal and atrophic muscles of the upper cervical spine', *Journal of Clinical Engineering*, Vol. 18, No. 5, pp. 433–9, 1993.

Hallgren, R., Greenman, P., Rechtien, J., 'Atrophy of suboccipital muscles in patients with chronic pain', *Journal of the American Osteopathic Association*, Vol. 94, No. 12, pp. 1032–8, 1994.

Hoefel, G., 'Effects of fasting on metabolism', *American Journal of Diseases in Children*, Vol. 28, pp. 16–24, 1928.

Hong, C., 'Difference in pain relief after trigger point injections in myofascial pain patients and without fibromyalgia', *Archives of Physical Medicine and Rehabilitation*, Vol. 77, No. 11, pp. 1161–6, November 1996.

'Hyperventilation and the anxiety state', editorial, *Journal of the Royal Society of Medicine*, Vol. 74, pp. 1–4, January, 1981.

Imamura, M., *et al.*, Trial of fasting on immunological reactions', *The Lancet*, pp. 760–3, 1958.

Jacobsen, S., *et al.*, 'Oral SAMe in primary fibromyalgia – a double blind clinical evaluation', *Scandinavian Journal of Rheumatology*, Vol. 20, No. 5, pp. 294–302, 1991.

Jameson, S., *et al.*, 'Pain relief and selenium balance in patients with connective tissue disease and osteoarthritis – a double blind study', *Nutrition Research Supplement*, Vol. 1, pp. 391–7, 1985.

Janda, V., 'Muscle and back pain – assessment and treatment', Physical Medicine Research Foundation Presentation, Montreal, 8–11 October, 1992.

Janda, Vladimir, 'Muscles and cervicogenic pain and syndromes', in *Physical Therapy of the Cervical and Thoracic Spine*, Grant, E. (ed.), Churchill Livingstone, London, pp. 153–66, 1988.

Janda,V., 'Muscle weakness and inhibition in back pain syndromes', in *Modern Manual Therapy of the Vertebral Column*, Grieve, Gregory (ed.), Churchill Livingstone, London, 1986.

Jiminez, C., *et al.*, 'Treatment of FMS with OMT and self-learned techniques', *Journal of the American Osteopathic Association*, Vol. 93, No. 8, p. 870, August 1993.

Jones, L., *Strain and Counterstrain*, American Academy of Osteopathy, Colorado Springs, 1981.

*Journal of Action for M.E.*, No. 15, spring, 1994.

Jull, Gwendolen, and Janda, Vladimir, 'Muscles and motor control in low back pain', in *Physical Therapy of the Low Back*, Twomey, Lance (ed.), pp. 253–78, Churchill Livingstone, London, 1987.

Kacera, W., 'Fibromyalgia and chronic fatigue – a different strain of the same disease?', *Canadian Journal of Herbalism*, Vol. XIV, No. IV, pp. 20–29, October, 1993.

Kalik, Joseph, 'Fibromyalgia: diagnosis and treatment of an important rheumatologic condition', *Journal of Osteopathic Medicine*, pp. 10–19, February, 1989.

Kamikawa, T., *et al.*, 'Effects of CoQ10 on exercise tolerance in chronic stable angina pectoris', *American Journal of Cardiology*, Vol. 56, No. 247, 1985.

Kenton, L., *Ageless Ageing*, Century Arrow, 1988.

Kernt, P., *et al.*, 'Fasting – pathophysiology and complications', *Western Journal of Medicine*, Vol. 137, pp. 379–99, 1982.

Keys, A., *Biology of Human Starvation*, Vols 1 and 2, University of Minnesota Press, 1950.

Kjeldsen-Kragh, J., *et al.*, 'Controlled trial of fasting and one-year vegetarian diet in rheumatoid arthritis', *The Lancet*, pp. 899–904, 1991.

Kraft, K., *et al.*, 'Reducing of pain in patients with fibromyalgia syndrome by applying a vibration massage device', *European Journal of Pain*, Supplement 5, pp. 15–295.

Kroker, G., 'Fasting and rheumatoid arthritis', *Clinical Ecology*, Vol. 2, No. 3, pp. 137–44, 1983.

Kleijnen, J., 'Ginkgo biloba', *The Lancet*, Vol. 340, No. 8828, pp. 1136–9, November, 1992.

Kobesova, A., *et al.*, 'Twenty-year-old pathogenic "active" postsurgical scar: a case study of a patient with persistent right lower quadrant pain', *Journal of Manipulative Physiological Therapy*, Vol. 30, pp. 234–238, 2007.

Kraft, K., *et al.*, 'Reducing of pain in patients with fibromyalgia syndrome by applying a vibration massage device', *European Journal of Pain*, Supplement 5, pp. 15–295, 2011.

Kwiat, G., 'Fibromyalgia and CFS linked to low vitamin $B_{12}$ and high homocysteine in CSF [cerebra-spinal fluid]', *Focus on Allergy Research*, pp. 1–2, May/June 1998.

Leventhal, L., 'FMS and parvovirus infection', *Arthritis and Rheumatism*, Vol. 34, pp. 1319–24, 1991.

Lewit, K., *Manipulation in Rehabilitation of the Locomotor System*, Butterworths, London, 1992.

Lowe, J., 'Metabolic rehabilitation of fibromyalgia patients', in Chaitow, L., *Fibromyalgia Syndrome – A practitioner's guide*, Churchill Livingstone, Edinburgh.

Lowe, J., *The Metabolic Treatment of Fibromyalgia*, Hawthorne BioMedical Press, Houston, 1997.

Lowe, J., *The Metabolic Treatment of Fibromyalgia*, McDowell Publishing Company, Tulsa, Oklahoma, 2000.

Lowe, J., *et al.*, 'Effectiveness and safety of T3 therapy for euthyroid fibromyalgia', *Clinical Bulletin of Myofascial Therapy*, Vol. 2, No. 2/3, pp. 31–58, 1997.

McCain, G., 'Role of physical fitness training in fibrositis/'fibromyalgia syndrome', *American Journal of Medicine*, Supplement 3A, pp. 73–7, 1986.

McEwan, B., 'The plasticity of the hippocampus is the reason for its vulnerability', *Seminars in Neuroscience*, Vol. 6, pp. 197–204, 1994.

Macintyre, A., 'What Causes M.E.? – The Immune Dysfunction Hypothesis', *Journal of Action for ME*, Vol. 14, pp. 24–5, 1993.

Martin *et al.*, 'An exercise program in treatment of fibromyalgia', *Journal of Rheumatology*, Vol. 23, No. 6, pp. 1050–3, June 1996.

Moldofsky, Harvey, 'Fibromyalgia, sleep disorder and chronic fatigue syndrome', Ciba Foundation Symposium 173, Chronic Fatigue Syndrome, pp. 262–79, Ciba, 1993.

Mose, J., 'Effects of echinacia on phagocytosis of NK cells', *Medical Welt*, Vol. 34, pp. 1463–7, 1983.

Nash, P., 'Chronic coxsackie B infection mimicking primary FMS', *Journal of Rheumatology*, Vol. 116, pp. 1506–8, 1989.

Niddam, D., *et al.*, 'Central representation of hyperalgesia from myofascial trigger point', *Neuroimage* 39, pp. 1299–1306, 2008.

Pizzorno, J., *Total Wellness*, Prima Publishing, Rocklin, California, 1996.

Pujol, J., *et al.*, 'Mapping brain response to pain in fibromyalgia patients using temporal analysis of FMRI', PLoS One 2009;4(4):e5224, 2009.

Rathbun, J., and Macnab, I., 'Microvascular patterns of the rotator cuff', *Journal of Bone and Joint Surgery*, Vol. 52, pp. 540–53, 1970.

Rothschild, Bruce, 'Fibromyalgia: an explanation for the aches and pains of the nineties', *Comprehensive Therapy*, Vol. 17, No. 6, pp. 9–14, 1991.

Rucco, V., *et al.*, 'Autogenic Training versus Erickson's analogical technique in treatment of fibromyalgia syndrome', *Rev. European Sci. Med. Farmacol*, Vol. 17, No. 1, pp. 41–50, 1995.

Sandford Kiser, R., *et al.*, 'Acupuncture relief of chronic pain syndrome correlates with increased plasma metenkephalin concentrations', *The Lancet*, Vol. ii, pp. 1394–6, 1983.

Sañudo, B., 'Aerobic Exercise Versus Combined Exercise Therapy in

Women with Fibromyalgia Syndrome: A Randomized Controlled Trial', *Archives Phys Med Rehabilitation*, Vol. 91, pp. 1838–1843, 2010.

Sapolsky, R., 'Hippocampal damage associated with prolonged glucocorticoid exposure in primates', *Journal of Neuroscience*, Vol. 10, pp. 2897–2902, 1990.

Schaffter, V., 'Double blind study of the hypoxia protective effect of standardised *Ginkgo biloba*', *Arzneim-Forsch*, Vol. 35, pp. 1283–6, 1985.

Selye, Hans, *The Stress of Life*, McGraw-Hill, 1980.

Simms, R., 'FMS in patients infected with HIV', *American Journal of Medicine*, Vol. 92, pp. 368–74, 1992.

Simons, David, and Travell, Janet, *Myofascial Pain and Dysfunction: The trigger point manual* (2nd edn; Vol. 1), Williams and Wilkins, Baltimore, 1998.

Simons, D. G., 'Myofascial pain syndromes due to trigger points', *Manual Medicine*, Vol. 1, pp. 67–71, 1985.

Sonkin, L., 'Endocrine disorders and muscle dysfunction', in Gelb, B. (ed.), *Clinical Management of Head , Neck and TMJ Pain and Dysfunction*, W. B. Saunders, Philadelphia, 1985.

Stoltz, A., 'Effects of OMT on the tender points of FMS', *Journal of American Osteopathic Association*, Vol. 93, No. 8, p. 866, August, 1993.

Travell, Janet, and Simons, David, *Myofascial Pain and Dysfunction: The trigger point manual*, Williams and Wilkins, Baltimore, 1983.

Tuncer, T., 'Primary fibromyalgia and allergy', *Clinical Rheumatology*, Vol. 16, No. 1, pp. 9–12, 1997.

Unpublished study reported in *Touch Therapy Times*, Vol. 5, No. 10, October, 1994.

Vanfraechem, J. H. P., 'CoQ10 and physical performance', *Biomedical and Clinical Aspects of CoQlO*,Vol. 3, pp. 235–41, 1981.

Van Why, R., Fibromyalgia and Massage Symposium, 1994.

Vorberg, G., 'Ginkgo extract – a longterm study of chronic cerebral insufficiency', *Clinical Trials Journal*, Vol. 22, pp. 149–57, 1985.

Wall, P., and Melzack, R., *Textbook of Pain*, Churchill Livingstone, London, 1989.

Warot, D., *et al.*, 'Comparative effects of Ginkgo biloba extracts on psychomotor performance and memory in healthy subjects', *Therapie*, No. 46, pp. 33–6, January–February, 1991.

Weindruch, R., and Walford, R., *Retardation of Aging and Disease by Dietary Restriction*, Charles Thomas, Springfield, Illinois, 1988.

Weinrech, S. P., *et al.*, 'Effects of massage on pain in cancer patients', *Applied Nursing Research*, Vol. 3, No. 4, pp. 140–5, 1990.

Werbach, M., *Nutritional Influences on Illness*, Third Line Press, Tarzana, California, 1991.

Wilke, S., 'Hypothyroidism with presenting symptoms of fibrositis', *Journal of Rheumatology*, Vol. 8, pp. 627–30, 1981.

Wing, E., 'Fasting enhanced immune effector mechanism', *American Journal of Medicine*, Vol. 75, pp. 91–6, 1983.

Wolf, F., 'Clinical syndrome of fibrositis' in *The Fibrositis/Fibromyalgia Syndrome*, Bennet, R. (ed.), *American Journal of Medicine*, 3A Supplement, No. 12, 1986.

Wolfe, F., 'The epierolology of tender points', *Journal of Rheumatology*, Vol. 12, No. 4, pp. 1164–8, 1985.

Wolfe, Frederick, Simons, David, *et al.*, 'The Fibromyalgia and myofascial pain syndromes', *Journal of Rheumatology*, Vol. 19, No. 6, pp. 944–51, 1992.

Yunus, M., 'Fibromyalgia and other functional syndromes', *Journal of Rheumatology*, Vol. 16, Supplement 19, No. 69, 1989.

## Further reading

Baldry, P.E., *Acupuncture Trigger Points and Musculoskeletal Pain*, Churchill Livingstone, London, 1993.

Block, Sidney, 'Fibromyalgia and the rheumatisms', *Controversies in Clinical Rheumatology*, Vol. 19, No. 1, pp. 61–78, February, 1993.

Boyle, W., Lectures in *Naturopathic Hydrotherapy*, O.H. Buckeye Press, East Palestine, 1991.

Cantu, R., Grodin, A., *Myofascial Manipulation*, Aspen Publications, Gaithersburg, Maryland, 1992.

Chaitow, L., *Candida Albicans*, Thorsons, 1995.

Chaitow, L. (Medical Ed.), 'Hydrotherapy', *Alternative Medicine*, Future

Medicine Publications, San Francisco, 1994.

Cott, A., *Fasting – the ultimate diet*, Bantam Books, New York, 1975.

Duna, George, 'Diagnosis, etiology and therapy of fibromyalgia', *Comprehensive Therapy*, Vol. 19, No. 2, pp. 60–3, 1993.

Ediger, Beth, *Coping with Fibromyalgia*, LRH Publications, Toronto, 1991.

Fibromyalgia Network Newsletter, pp. 3–5, April, 1993 (report on tests for fibromyalgia).

Fibromyalgia Network Newsletters, Compendium 2, pp. 48–9 (report on 2nd Los Angeles Chronic Fatigue and Immune Deficit Syndrome Conference, May 18/19, 1991).

Fibromyalgia Network Newsletters, October 1990 to January 1992, Compendium 2, January 1993, May 1993, Compendium, January 1994, July 1994.

Fishbain, David, 'Diagnosis of patients with myofascial pain syndrome', *Archives of Physical and Medical Rehabilitation*, Vol. 70, pp. 433–8, June, 1989.

Goldenberg, Don, 'Fibromyalgia, chronic fatigue syndrome and myofascial pain syndrome', *Current Opinions in Rheumatology*, Vol. 5, pp. 199–208, 1993.

Jacobsen, Soren, 'Dynamic muscular endurance in primary fibromyalgia compared with chronic myofascial pain syndrome', *Archives of Physical and Medical Rehabilitation*, Vol. 73, pp. 170–3, February, 1992.

Jevning, R., 'The physiology of meditation – a wakeful hypometabolic integrated response', *Neuroscience and Biobehavioural Reviews*, Vol. 16, pp. 415–24, 1992.

*Journal of Action for ME*, No. 15, spring, 1994.

Kaada, B., *et al.*, 'Increase in plasma beta-endorphins in connective tissue massage', *General Pharmacology*, Vol. 20, No.4, pp. 487–9, 1989.

Levin, S., *Massage Effects on Stress Response,* thesis, University of North Carolina, Greensboro, 1990.

Maryon, Francis, 'Fibrositis (fibromyalgia syndrome) and the dental clinician', *Journal of Craniomandibular Practice*, Vol. 9, No. 1, pp. 64–70, January, 1991.

Melzack, R., *et al.*, 'Pain mechanisms-a new theory', *Science*, Vol. 150, pp.

971–9, 1965.

*Physiotherapy*, Vol. 76, No. 4, pp. 207–10, April, 1990.

Pizzorno, J., and Murray, M. (eds), 'Hydrotherapy' in *Textbook of Natural Medicine*, Bastyr University, Seattle, 1989.

Readhead, C., 'Enhanced adaptive behavioural response in patients pre-treated by breathing retraining', *The Lancet*, pp. 665–8, 22 September, 1984.

Rubin, B., *et al.*, 'Treatment options in fibromyalgia syndrome', *Journal of American Osteopathic Association*, Vol. 90, No. 9, pp. 844–5, September, 1990.

Salloum, T., 'Fasting' in *Textbook of Natural Medicine*, Pizzorno, J., and Murray, M. (eds), Bastyr University, Seattle, 1989.

Scott, J.T., *Arthritis and Rheumatism*, Oxford University Press, Oxford, 1980.

Simons, D., 'Fibrositis/fibromyalgia – a form of myofascial trigger points?', *American Journal of Medicine*, Vol. 81, Supplement 3A, pp. 93–8, 19.

# Useful Publications and Addresses

## Publications

*The CFIDS Chronicle*
PO Box 220398
Charlotte, NC 28222-0398

*Fibromyalgia Network*
A quarterly newsletter for
fibromyalgia, fibrositis and
chronic fatigue syndrome support
groups, available from:
PO Box 31750
Tucson, AZ 85751-1750
Tel: (520) 290-5508
(800) 853-2929
http://www.fmnetnews.com
https://www.facebook.com/
FibroNetwork

*Interaction*
Journal of Action for ME (three
issues a year), available from:
Action for ME

42 Temple Street, Keynsham,
Bristol BS31 1EH, England
http://www.actionforme.org.
uk/get-informed/publications/
interaction-magazine/latest-ia-
issue

*CAM*
A magazine for complementary
and alternative practitioners
Website: http://www.cam-mag.com

*Journal of Bodywork and
Movement Therapies*
Website:http://www.harcourt
international .com/journals/jbmt

*The Update*
available from: Massachusetts
CFIDS Association
808 Main St
Waltham, MA 02154
(617) 893-4415

Mass CFIDS/ME & FM
Association
P.O. Box 690305
Quincy, MA 02269-0305, USA
https://www.masscfids.
org/newsletter/sign-up-for-newsletter

## Support Groups

### CANADA
Association Québécoise de la
Fibromyalgie
333 boul. Lacombe, suite 208
LeGardeur (Quebec) J5Z 1N2

ME FM Societies of British
Columbia
Box 462
Vancouver BC V5Z 1K7
http://www.mefm.bc.ca

FM-CFS Canada
For support groups and help
throughout Canada, visit the
FM-CFS Canada website.
Resources in English and French.
www.fm-cfs.ca

Ontario Fibrositis Association
c/o Arthritis Society
393 University Avenue,
Suite 1700
Toronto, ON M5G 1E6
www.arthritis.ca

### HOLLAND
Fibromyalgia: Eendrachtic Sterk
A. Reijnderstraat B235
9663 PN Pekele

### INTERNATIONAL ASSOCIATION FOR CFS/ME
27 N. Wacker Drive, Suite 416
Chicago, IL, 60606
*Tel*: (847) 258-7248
http://www.asafund.org/resource.htm

### MEN WITH FIBROMYALGIA
www.menwithfibro.com

### NORWAY
Norsk Fibrositt Forbund
Oksenøystien 4
1324 Lysaker

### UNITED KINGDOM
Action for ME
42 Temple Street, Keynsham,
Bristol BS31 1EH
Tel: 0117 927 9551
http://www.actionforme.org.uk

Fibromyalgia Association
PO Box 206
Stourbridge
West Midlands DY9 8YL
*Tel*: 01384 820052
*Fax*: 01834 869467
*email*: fms@cableinet.co.uk

The main body for details
regarding various support groups
in the UK

The Centre for Fibromyalgia (UK)
Bascombe Manor Medical Centre
40 Florence Road, Bournemouth
Dorset BH5 1HQ
*Tel:* 01202 303012 or 01202 303013
Website: www.ukfibromyalgia.com

Leon Chaitow ND DO Senior Lecturer
University of Westminster
Practice details: http://www.
IntegrativeHealthcare. co.uk
Appointments: 020 7486 6664

– or –

PO Box 41
Corfu
Greece 49100
Fax: 00 30 661 97716
Book details and on-line
interview: Website: http://www.
harcourt international.com/
chaitow

*Journal of Bodywork and Movement Therapies* details/
articles: http://www.journals.
elsevier.com/journal-of-
bodywork-and-movement-
therapies/

## USA

Arthritis Foundation
1330 W. Peachtree, Suite 100
Atlanta, GA 30309
*Tel:* (404) 872-7100
http://www.arthritis.org/
arthritis-facts/disease-center/
fibromyalgia.php

The CFIDS Association of
America (for chronic fatigue and
immune dysfunction)
PO Box 223098
Charlotte, NC 28222-0398

Fibromyalgia Alliance of America
PO Box 21990
Columbus, OH 43221-0990

Fibromyalgia Association of
Greater Washington
13203 Valley Drive
Woodbridge, VA 22191-1531

Fibromyalgia Association of
Texas
5650 Forest Lane
Dallas, TX 75230

Fibromyalgia Information
Foundation
PO Box 19016
Portland, OR 97280
Website: www.myalgia.com

Fibromyalgia Network
5700 Stockdale Hwy #100
Bakersfield, CA 93309
*Tel:* (415) 541-5075

Fibromyalgia Support Groups of
New Hampshire
c/o Arthritis Foundation NH
6 Chenell Drive
Concord, NH 03301-9322
*Tel:* (603) 224-9322

Gulf Coast CFID/CFS Association
752 J Avenue Estancias
Venice, FL 34292-2316
*Tel*: (813) 548-8237

National Fibromyalgia Association
2121 S. Towne Centre Place
Suite 300
Anaheim, CA 92806
*Tel*: (714) 921-0150
*Fax*: (714) 921-6920
http://www.fmaware.org

Fibromyalgia Seattle
19655 1st Ave. So. Ste. 205
Normandy Park, WA 98148
www.discussfibromyalgia.com

Fundamental Physiology LLC
Website: http://www.
drginahoneyman.com/
Dr. Gina Honeyman-Lowe
2525 Arapahoe Avenue, E4-308
Boulder, CO 80302
*Tel*: 303.413.9100
*Fax*: 1.888.728.3490

Southern California CFIDS
Network
23732 Hillhurst Drive Number 9
Laguna Niguel, CA 92677
*Tel*: (714) 249-6976

WebMD
www.webmd.com/fibromyalgia/
guide/fibromyalgia-resources-
index

## Diagnostic tests

### UNITED KINGDOM

Health Interlink
Interlink House
22 Digby Drive
Leicestershire Rd
Melton Mowbray
Leicestershire LE13 0RQ
Tel: 01664 562454
www.health-interlink.com
Note: practitioner needs to make
contact, not patient

BioLab
Stone House
9 Weymouth Street
London W1W 6DB
Tel: 0207 636 5959
Note : on referral from doctor
only

### USA

Genova Diagnostics
63 Zillicoa Street
Ashville, NC 28810-1074
Tel: 01 828-253-0621
Website: http:/ /www.gdx.net

# Index

essential (omega-6) fatty acids 156, 158, 246

essential oils 142-4

exclusion and rotation diets 125-9

exercise 7, 96, 101, 209-13, 226, 227, 231-3, 248, 249

extremities, cold 16 *see also* Raynaud's phenomenon

eye imbalances 84-5

eye movements 212

eyes, dry 3, 45

facilitation 90-2, 103, 111, 191

fascia 83-4

fasting 161, 163, 173-4

fatigue 2, 6, 7, 16, 25, 29, 30, 38-40, 96, 249

   treatment 148-50

feet

   numbness/tingling 6, 42

   swollen feeling 2

Felson, D. 225-6

fever, low-grade 11, 39

Fibromyalgia Network 13, 20-2

fibrosis 87

fibrositis 6, 12, 150, 238

fish oils 152

flexibility 210

   exercises 232

'flotation tanks' 174

food intolerance questionnaire 126-8

frontal lobe activity 107

gas (wind) 18

'generalized rheumatism' 225, 226

*Giardia lamblia* 42, 154

*Ginkgo biloba* 117, 155, 236-8, 248

Glucose Tolerance Factor 150

goitrogens 159

Goldenberg, Don 9, 10, 11-12, 46, 57, 225-6

Goldstein, Jay 107, 110, 113-14, 120

Greenman, P. 103

Grodin, Alan 224

group treatment 235-6

growth hormone 108

   low levels 79, 104, 120

   sleep and 48, 100

   stimulation 145, 161, 245

hair loss 3

Hallgreen, R. 103

hands

   numbness/tingling 6, 42, 64

   swollen feeling 2

Hauser, Gunnar 24

hay fever 22, 128

headaches 2, 6, 7, 16, 19, 20, 28, 30, 40-1, 95, 107

heart problems 41

heartburn 18

herbal medicine 236-8, 248

heterostasis 119-20

HHV6 (herpes virus) 59

hippocampus 109

histamine 29

HIV 58

homeopathy 126, 238-40, 248

homeostasis (self-healing) x-xiii, 110, 116, 119-24, 179, 227-8

homocysteine 245

hormonal imbalance 63, 94, 108-9, 115, 120

hydrotherapy 141-2, 174-S, 248

hyperhydration, premenstrual 157-8

hyperthyroidism 65

hyperventilation 27-33, 83, 112, 113, 115, 134, 181 *see also* breathing exercises

hypnotherapy 240

hypothalamic-pituitary-adrenal axis 108

hypothalamus 109

hypothyroidism 53, 65

immune dysfunction model 24

immune system 48, 110, 114, 119

   depression/disturbance 24, 44, 50, 57, 80, 120

   enhancing 58, 74, 122, 176, 179

immunizations 44

indigestion 30

infections xi, 18, 20, 76 *see also* bacteria; parasites; viral infections; yeast infections

inflammation x, 12, 78, 143

   treatment 150-4

injections, trigger points 231, 236

injury 3, 20, 105 *see also* whiplash

iodine 159

iron deficiency 75, 94, 148, 159

irritability 3

irritable bowel syndrome 2, 6-7, 7, 18, 19, 20, 25, 41-2, 96

   treatment 154-5

ischemia (hypoxia) 86, 100, 100, 237

Jessop, Carol 15-17, 17-18, 34, 44, 56

joints, hypermobile ('loose ligaments') 8, 41, 80, 84, 212

Kakkar, Vijay 175

Keppler, R. 243

*Klebsiella* 46, 61

*L. bulgaricus* 154

lavender essential oil 143-4

lead toxicity 157

'leaky gut syndrome' 35

leukotrienes 151

limbic system 24, 43, 109-13

liver support 160, 162

'loose ligaments' see joints, hypermobile

Lowe, John 54, 64, 65, 66

lupus erythematosus 67

Lyme disease 3, 62

lymph glands, swollen 11, 17, 39

lysine 169

Macintyre, Anne 23, 57

magnesium 17,46, 64, 144, 148, 157, 244, 245

magnetic resonance imaging (MRI) 77, 103

malic acid 244

massage 178, 205-9, 240-1, 248

ME Action 13, 23

medication 241-2, 248, 249

melatonin 144, 246

Melzack, R. 94, 97

memory problems 3, 16, 21, 24, 106, 107, 155-6, 237

Mena, Ismael 111

menopause 63, 143-4, 175
mental calm 134
migraine 40
mitral valve prolapse 19, 41
Moldofsky, Harvey 11, 49, 51
monodiet 163-4
mood swings 3
morning stiffness 2, 7, 96
Mountz, James 107
mouth, dry 3, 16, 45
mouth ulcers 3
multiple sclerosis (MS) 68, 77
muscle energy treatment 186-90,
   204-5, 211, 248
muscle enzyme assessments 78
muscle relaxants 242
muscles
   effects of sleep disturbance
   49, 100
   in fibromyalgia 100-4
   'micro-trauma' 101, 104
   normal and abnormal pain 83
   reaction to stress 82-100
   twitching 16
   weak (inhibited) 212
muscular dystrophy 77
muscular release 134
myalgic encephalomyelitis (ME)
   see chronic fatigue syndrome
myoclonus (restless leg
   syndrome) 3, 7, 19, 51
myofascial pain syndrome (MPS)
   11, 55, 94-7, 99, 105, 190,
   192, 229, 247
myofascial release techniques
   223-4
myofascial trigger points see
   trigger points

nails, white spots 16
names of conditions, confusion
   and importance 10-13
narcotics 227
natural killer cells 80, 120
neck
   pain 29, 181
   tenderness 17
neroli essential oil 144
neuropathy 68
neurotransmitters 50, 109, 115
   imbalances 79
neutral baths 141-2, 174, 248
neutral (dummy) points 5
night cramps 3
nutritional deficiencies 17-18,
   148
nutritional evaluation tests 77
nutritional supplementation
   244-6, 248
   sleep problems 144-5

Oligoantigenic diet 129-32
ornithine 145, 245
osteoarthritis 3, 20, 62
osteopathy 69, 180, 181, 214,
   242-4, 249
overuse syndrome 68

pain 6, 11, 21
   brain regulation 24, 107
   nutritional treatment 150-4
   sensitivity see substance P
   tolerance overload 115
   widespread 4, 7
   see also tender points; trigger
   points
pain relief 180-1
   exercise 209-13, 231-3

self-massage 205-9
Selye, Hans 119
serotonin 33, 38, 45, 50, 79, 100, 109, 145, 241, 245
Sicca syndrome 3, 45
side-effects 171-2
silicone breast implant syndrome 3, 46
*Silybum marianum* 162, 165
Simms, R. 5, 58
Simons, David 55, 93, 99, 101
single photon emission computerized tomography (SPECT) scans 33, 40, 103, 107, 107, 111
Sjögren's syndrome 73
skin, itchy 3
skin brushing 166-7
skipping 210
sleep apnoea 3, 50
sleep problems 2, 6, 8--9, 16, 18, 21, 27, 30, 39, 47-52, 78, 96, 100
   treatment 132-46
sleep process 47-8
somatization 72
St John'sWort 38
steroid medication 34, 35, 67, 70, 227, 242
stool analysis 35, 77
Stotz, A. 243
strain-counterstrain methods 178-9, 182-6, 190, 211, 248
   tender points 214-24
stress xi-xii, 40, 119, 192
   effects on brain 113-14
   and hyperventilation 28-31
   reaction of muscles 82-100
   and toxic build-up 160

stretching 210, 248
substance abuse 3
substance P 32, 79, 100, 108, 109
sugar-rich diet 34, 115
supplementation *see* nutritional supplementation
support groups 248
surgery 20
swimming 210, 212, 231
sympathetic nervous system 72, 100, 132, 173
symptoms 2-8, 15-23

T'ai chi 210, 248
tapping 202
tempero-mandibular joint (TMJ) syndrome 19, 68-69
temporal arteritis 70
tender points 4-6, 16, 97, 98-99, 105
   locations 214-15
   treatment 182-6, 216--24, 241, 243
tendons 87
tennis ball massage 209
TENS treatment 240
thermo-regulatory hydrotherapy (TRH) 175-8
thermography 78
thermo-regulatory set point 120
throat, sore 11, 16, 39
thumb work 209
thyroid
   blood tests 52, 65, 75
   'cellular resistance' 52, 53, 54
   disease 20
   dysfunction 17, 24, 52-6, 66-8, 108, 111, 112, 113
   support 158-9

tiredness *see* fatigue
toxicity 24-5, 53, 114
treatment *see* detoxification
trampolining 210
tranquillizers 227
Travell, Janet 55, 93, 97, 101
trigger points 6, 29, 40, 55, 59,
    68-69, 72, 78, 81, 98-99, 105,
    247
    as cause of fibromyalgia 94-7
    development 93-4
    dry needling and injection 236
    finding and treating 191-209
    facilitation 92
    scars and 170
    summary of characterisitics
    97-9
    xylocaine injection 231
tryptophan 45, 79, 144, 245

Ultra-Clear 165
urethral pain 19
urination, frequent 16

vacations 227
Van Why, Richard 241
vibrational massage 241
viral infections 3, 50, 57-58, 73,
    94, 115
    treatment 169
visualizing movements 211
vitamins
    A 145, 158, 159
    B-complex 53, 55, 66, 94, 111,
    159, 246
    $B_3$ 245
    $B_5$ 148, 165
    $B_6$ 45, 64, 148, 156, 158, 245
    $B_{12}$ 245

C 94, 145, 146, 148, 159, 165,
    244, 246
E 51, 145, 146, 158, 244
folic acid 51, 148

walking 210, 212, 231
Wall, P. 94
Wallace, Daniel 51
weather sensitivity 2, 6, 95
Werbach, Melvyn 148
whiplash injury 58, 102-4
Wolf, F. 226
Wolfe, Frederick 99

x-rays 76

yeast (candida) infections 17, 34-
    7, 42, 44, 46, 94, 115, 154
    as cause of allergies 25-6
    sugar-loading test 35, 77
    treatment 146-7
yoga 210, 248
Yunus, Muhammad 5, 27-8, 108

zinc 17, 146, 159, 246